The End of the Obesity Epidemic

D0219745

Despite apocalyptic predictions from a vocal alliance of health professionals, politicians and social commentators that rising obesity levels would lead to a global health crisis, the crisis has not materialised. In this provocative follow-up to his classic work of obesity scepticism, *The Obesity Epidemic*, Michael Gard argues that we have entered into a new, and perhaps terminal, phase of the obesity debate.

Evidence suggests that obesity rates are levelling off in Western societies, life expectancies continue to rise in line with rising obesity rates, and across the world policy-makers have remained largely indifferent and inactive in the face of this apparently deadly threat to our health and well-being. Dissecting and dismissing much of the over-blown rhetoric and ideological bias found on both sides of the obesity debate, Gard demonstrates that the science of obesity remains radically uncertain and that it is impossible to establish an objective 'truth' on which to base policy. His powerful and inescapable conclusion is that we should now mark the end of the obesity epidemic.

Offering a road map through the maze of claims and counter-claims, while still holding to a sceptical standpoint, this book provides an unparalleled anatomy of obesity as a scientific, political and cultural issue. It is essential reading for anybody with an interest in the science or sociology of health and lifestyle.

Michael Gard is Associate Professor in the Faculty of Education at Charles Sturt University's Bathurst campus. He teaches and writes about health, physical education, sport and the media and is a regular media commentator on these topics. His previous work in this field includes his book *The Obesity Epidemic: Science, Morality and Ideology*, co-written with Jan Wright.

The End of the Obesity Epidemic

Michael Gard

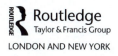
Routledge
Taylor & Francis Group

LONDON AND NEW YORK

First published 2011
by Routledge
2 Park Square, Milton Park, Abingdon, Oxon, OX14 4RN

Simultaneously published in the USA and Canada
by Routledge
270 Madison Avenue, New York, NY 10016

Routledge is an imprint of the Taylor & Francis Group, an informa business

Typeset in Times New Roman by Swales & Willis Ltd, Exeter, Devon
Printed and bound in Great Britain by
CPI Antony Rowe, Chippenham, Wiltshire

British Library Cataloguing in Publication Data
A catalogue record for this book is available from the British Library

Library of Congress Cataloging-in-Publication Data
Gard, Michael, 1965–
    The end of the obesity epidemic / by Michael Gard.
        p.; cm.
    1. Obesity—Epidemiology. 2. Obesity—Social aspects. I. Title.
    [DNLM: 1. Obesity—epidemiology. 2. Obesity—psychology. WD 210 G217e 2011]
    RA645.O23G366 2011
    362.196'398—dc22
    2010018103

ISBN 13: 978–0–415–48987–4 hbk
ISBN 13: 978–0–415–48988–1 pbk
ISBN 13: 978–0–203–88119–4 ebk

To Beverly Margaret Gard, my mother, whose bravery, toughness and beauty will live with me for ever.

Contents

List of figures

List of tables

Acknowledgements

Small sections of this book, distributed across a number of chapters, were previously published in:

Gard, M. (2009) 'Friends, enemies and the cultural politics of critical obesity research', in: J. Wright and V. Harwood (eds) *Biopolitics and the 'Obesity Epidemic': Governing Bodies*, New York: Routledge: 31–44.

Following the publication of *The Obesity Epidemic: Science, Morality and Ideology*, my co-author and I were ridiculed for not publishing our work in the mainstream medical journals. Apparently this was meant to cast doubt on the quality of our ideas. This was perhaps understandable but, still, a serious mistake, not least because my co-author was Jan Wright, a formidable researcher and thinker in any company. Although not an author here, Jan remains a friend and colleague and read large sections of this book while it was being written. Regardless of its final merits, it is a different and better book because of her advice.

I was also fortunate to have been able to correspond with Tim Olds during this project. Tim read and commented on Chapter 3 and has been a patient and insightful correspondent. In an age where many academics compete for prestige, he combines rare talent with exemplary generosity. Thanks also to Carolyn Vander Schee for her virtual and non-virtual companionship over a long period of time and for kindly agreeing to co-author Chapter 5 of this book. Carolyn has been my collaborator and 'skipper' on a number of obesity-related research projects, an intellectual ally and close friend.

This book was helped along by a few self-appointed though criminally under-paid research assistants, who cut out newspaper columns and dropped them in my pigeonhole or emailed me news stories and references. Foremost amongst these was my Charles Sturt University colleague Rylee Dionigi, another incurably generous spirit and cherished friend. Darren Powell from New Zealand also passed on some particularly useful material.

Other friends and colleagues listened patiently as I waffled on about the end of the obesity epidemic and offered their own intelligent comments and suggestions. They include Jo Morin, Sarah Howard, Lisette Burrows, Mark Falcous, John Evans, Emma Rich, Kirsten Bell and Alan Bain.

I want to particularly thank the University of Otago and its School of Physical Education, who supported my travel to New Zealand in early 2010 and gave me the opportunity to test-run some of my ideas at their 'Big Fat Truth' conference. I also received generous support from the Centre for Appearance Research at the University of Western England to attend 'Size Matters?' in June 2009 and from the University of British Columbia's Department of Anthropology for their conference 'Alcohol, Tobacco and Obesity: Deconstructing the New Public Health's Axis of Evil' in July of 2009. In between these two conferences, Symeon Dagkas and Richard Bailey hosted me on a brief but hugely enjoyable visit to the University of Birmingham, where I presented and discussed some of the research contained in this book.

As ever, my own institution Charles Sturt University and its School of Human Movement Studies have been a constant support, now stretching back over fourteen years. In this respect, the guidance and friendship of my department head, Frank Marino, stand out above all others. Some debts of gratitude are so great that it is pointless to try to explain them. Suffice to say that Frank and his family have lived the highs and lows of my life in Bathurst and there is a chair in heaven for each one of them.

In June 2010 I left Bathurst to be nearer my parents, Ralph and Beverly. I want to acknowledge my extended Bathurst family for all they have given me and for each playing a part in creating the perfect working and living environment. Thanks to Rod Allan, Joan Philip, Jo Reid, Bill Green, Lucy Zundans, Greg Fraser, Jane Mitchell, Tim Roebuck, Cal Abbott, Spud Murphy and many others. Thanks also to the staff of Bathurst's best cafes, The Hub, Al Dente and Le Gall, where a sizeable portion of this book was written.

Not much of what I do these days happens when or in the way I initially imagined and this puts great pressure on those who work with me. The staff at Taylor & Francis have once again been supportive and reasonable in all my dealings with them. Thanks to Simon Whitmore, Joshua Wells, Brian Guerin and their colleagues for all their patience and understanding.

To my parents, our journey together continues to take many unexpected and, in a few cases, painful twists and turns. Through it all, you have given me something that everyone needs but only a few can give: unconditional love and a place to belong.

1 The beginning is the end

An obituary

The obesity epidemic was born some time around the year 2000 and died about ten years later. Many tried to revive it and convince themselves that the situation was not terminal, but by the end of the first decade of the twenty-first century there was nothing that could be done. This book is, in part, a small contribution to the history of the obesity epidemic's short but spectacular life.

It is true that it had been prophesied during the preceding 100 years. The prophets included physicians, surgeons, epidemiologists and insurance salesmen, each with a barrow to push, something to sell or sometimes both. Their confidence about the looming crisis grew as people really did get fatter during the second half of the twentieth century. Trouble was, no one seemed to be listening.

By the turn of the new century the obesity prophets were prepared to wait no longer. They decided that the moment of crisis had arrived and so the obesity epidemic was created, more or less, with the purpose of getting people to sit up and take notice. There was nothing special about the year 2000; obesity rates did not hit a magical number, the number of obesity-related deaths had not changed (in fact no one knew how many obesity-related deaths there were or, really, what an obesity-related death actually was) and life expectancies were still rising steadily in the parts of the world we might have expected them to rise. In fact, on many measures most people were healthier than ever before.

What changed around 2000 was the rhetoric. Almost overnight, obesity joined the ranks of famous infectious contagions and was transformed from a slow-moving inconvenience into an agile killer. Apparently respectable medical researchers attempted to make the argument that it spread from person to person and, given time, would reduce life expectancies and match the devastation of plagues, terrorist bombs, rising sea levels and mass species extinction. As an epidemic, obesity now moved in totally new rhetorical circles. A simple twist in the language catapulted it out of the medical B grade, occupied by the likes of toenail fungus and back pain, and into the big league alongside AIDS, cancer and heart disease.

But just as the light from the sun reaches us eight minutes after its emission, the prophets of the obesity epidemic could not know that the object of their fascination was already nothing more than an echo of the past. They talked of a world in which obesity rates were not only increasing, but increasing at an increasing rate. They were wrong, but the word 'exponential' continued to be thrown around in scientific journals and newspapers alike – a perplexing situation that the language of 'epidemic' no doubt helped to facilitate.

Towards the end of the first decade of the new century the cracks of doubt began to appear. The ranks of the non-believers were slowly swelling and reports from around the world suggested that not only was the year 2000 the beginning of the obesity epidemic as an idea, it was probably also close to the moment when it, quite literally, began to die. The beginning, as it were, was the end.

As is often the case when new crises are unearthed in the media, early press coverage of the obesity epidemic lurched from alarm to hysteria. In Australia, fresh from unprecedented success at the 2000 Sydney Olympics, it was seriously suggested in the months following the games that rising childhood obesity might drain the nation's talent pool and jeopardise its cherished record of international sporting success. It seemed to occur to no one that, if nothing else, childhood obesity was on the rise in most of the countries that were inclined to invest heavily in sport. So while we might wonder whether there is any connection at all between childhood obesity rates and elite sporting success, there was as least the comfort that we were all in the same boat.

The silliness of this example was enough to pique my interest in the kinds of concerns that increasing obesity rates were beginning to generate. At the time I knew that obesity had been rising for decades and that the lack of concerted government action had long frustrated some epidemiologists and health researchers. What had changed? Why was the issue now gaining the traction that had eluded it for so long?

My colleague Jan Wright and I decided to follow the growing outcry. We had a number of motivations. We knew that many of the more serious claims being made in scientific journals and the media were simply mistaken. For example, it was inaccurate to claim, as many repeatedly did, that modern children were less physically active than the children of previous generations. Very little compelling scientific evidence to support this idea had ever existed and, as I show later in this book, a number of scientists have recently and publicly recanted their previous statements on this subject.

Jan and I could also see that the idea of an obesity epidemic was likely to have unpredictable and even dangerous effects in the world. As physical educators, the potential for unnecessary, ineffective and unethical things being done to children in schools seemed obvious to us. This too is a matter to which I return with the luxury of greater historical perspective in this book.

Finally, our work also contributed to a small but growing research literature that questioned the medical significance of rising body weights. While it could scarcely be doubted that more fat people would have some impact on the rates of some diseases, there were serious questions to be asked about the nature and size of these impacts. Was it possible, for example, that the language of 'crisis' and 'epidemic' made it much more difficult to get a handle on what we might call the 'real' or 'objective' impact of rising obesity? In other words, did the new hyperbolic rhetorical landscape make it harder to mount a rational and proportional response to the problem? Might it lead to resources being channelled in directions where they simply were not needed, while reducing support for more appropriate and cost-effective interventions?

Our research into the issue culminated in 2005 with the publication of *The Obesity Epidemic: Science, Morality and Ideology* (Gard and Wright 2005). Since then, the obesity epidemic has continued on its remarkable journey, turning up in both expected and unexpected places. This book is partly an attempt to update and build upon the questions raised and claims made in *The Obesity Epidemic* in the context of this journey. But it also an attempt to take stock of the last ten years and to understand why the obesity epidemic started, how it ended and what lessons we might learn.

Towards a history

I tried to keep two kinds of readers in mind while writing this book. The first has a general interest in obesity, perhaps perplexed or intrigued by the book's title, but not intimately familiar with the obesity literature or the debates that have accompanied it. But I have also attempted to engage with readers who know a great deal about the subject, may even have read *The Obesity Epidemic* and are able to contextualise the research presented in these pages for themselves. In other words, I was confronted with a challenge familiar to many writers of non-fiction; I was anxious not to confuse the first kind of reader by taking too much for granted while not wanting to patronise or bore the second.

I have approached this challenge in two ways. First, where I judged that knowing the context was important to understanding the arguments I was trying to make, I have provided this context. As a result, this book is, in part, a kind of history of the obesity epidemic, albeit a partisan history, written from my own highly interested point of view. I am not so much concerned here with trying to persuade readers as I am with telling a story about the study of obesity. Yes, I will offer readers the truth about obesity as I see it and yes, I do think that in 2010 we are at the beginning of the end of the obesity epidemic. But my hope is that readers will get a great deal more from this book than my assessment of the current state of research. In particular, I have tried to paint a picture of the various participants in debates about obesity and to leave the reader with an expanded sense of where and why there is so much disagreement in this field of study.

A second feature of this book is perhaps more contentious and may even trouble some readers. This is a more personal book than *The Obesity Epidemic*. It is personal because, as well as being a producer of knowledge about obesity, my work over the last decade has involved publicly advocating for certain points of view. This means that I have been interviewed, written for newspapers and, perhaps as a result, been criticised and vilified on air and in public. In my experience it is much easier to make controversial arguments in the safety of the pages of academic journals or the university seminar room than it is in front of a live-radio microphone or in a 600-word newspaper article. The process of trying to combine scholarship and advocacy has forced me to reflect constantly on the kinds of arguments I have made and to ask myself 'Do I really believe the things I say and write?'

So, particularly with the second kind of reader in mind, I have attempted to tell a second story about the evolution of my thinking about the study of obesity. Lest this be taken to be an unforgivable self-indulgence, let me offer a little background.

Beginning around the turn of the century, the initial explosion of publicity surrounding the obesity epidemic was led by a broad coalition of scientists, epidemiologists and medical researchers, later amplified by journalists, politicians and many other interest groups. Not surprisingly, the sheer volume and intensity of obesity rhetoric gave rise to an opposing point of view: were rising obesity levels *really* the mother of all public health catastrophes? My initial work with Jan Wright was part of a small but impassioned, mostly academic movement that sought to dispute obesity epidemic rhetoric. Rather than epidemiologists and medical researchers, my colleagues in this enterprise were drawn mostly from the social sciences. In short, the emerging landscape was one consisting of a mostly all-powerful alarmist Goliath (them) and a tiny, largely peripheral and sceptical David (us). It would therefore be possible to characterise the last ten years of obesity research as a case of two opposing, if unevenly matched, combatants.

And yet, this characterisation would be inaccurate. In reality, debates about obesity are far more complex and multi-layered than the two-camps picture might suggest. A little digging shows that alarmists and sceptics vary hugely. So as well as trying to offer a guided tour of this complexity, I attempt in this book to steer a path through the opposing arguments and to offer an analysis of the obesity epidemic that is beholden to no camp. In particular, my position as an obesity sceptic has evolved so that I am now inclined to pose questions about the thinking of people on all sides of the debate, not just alarmists. I do this partly because of some dissatisfaction with the arguments made by those whom I would once have seen (and mostly still do see) as my intellectual allies. More important, though, my goal here is to offer the first (to my knowledge) attempt to read the obesity epidemic from both sides of the debate. I do not claim that this reading is exhaustive; no doubt others are in the pipeline. However, my modest hope here is to challenge even experienced readers of obesity research; I hope to provoke them into agreeing or disagreeing with me or, at the very least, thinking again about their own beliefs and assumptions.

In short, this book is an attempt to begin the process of writing the history of the obesity epidemic and the way people have chosen to think about it. Some will see this as profoundly misguided or at least naively premature. My response in this book is to argue that whatever happens in the following decades, by 2010 a new phase in the obesity epidemic had been reached, marking the end of a period of consciousness raising or hyperbole (depending on your point of view) and a transitioning into something else. Whether the future will deliver waxing or waning rhetoric about the obesity time-bomb is unclear. What I think we can say with more certainty is that the obesity research community has managed to convince a significant percentage of the population that they should think and worry a great deal about their own and other people's body weight. The monumental task of educating the planet is largely complete. The question now is 'What next?'

Friend or enemy?

My final reason for writing this book was, for me at least, the most important and thought provoking. Let me illustrate by quoting from two customer reviews of *The Obesity Epidemic* taken from Amazon.com, the first mostly complimentary, the second much more critical.

> This book takes a look at a variety of obesity research with a fresh eye. It assumes nothing, and what is revealed with this unbiased eye will surprise and amaze most readers. As many know, diets don't work. This helps explain why fat people aren't fat due to gluttony.
>
> (customer review, Amazon.com)

> The authors argue that because science has not solved the complexities of body weight regulation today it never will. And furthermore, that even if it could, people's thinking about body weight would never change. Surely, this is too rigid thinking. It is like saying that because physics has not come up with a grand unifying theory today, all physics research is useless and it won't make any progress in the future. Or that because we can't cure Parkinson's disease now, we never will. This is unacceptable on its face. Also untrue is that people's perceptions and actions do not change. In the days before Prozac, depression was poorly understood and treated; after Prozac the public, health care professionals and others came to see that at least some depression was a neurochemical imbalance. The sudden swings in the public's eating habits, such as the low-carb phenomenon, is further testament to the power of the public to seek out and employ hopeful approaches to weight control.
>
> (customer review, Amazon.com)

For the first reviewer, *The Obesity Epidemic* was 'unbiased' and 'assumes nothing' while, for the second, it was a rigid and premeditated attack on scientific progress. The generation of such diametrically opposing reactions is probably neither surprising nor, in my view, a bad thing. The important point for me, though, is what appear to be the reasons behind these interpretations.

The first reviewer seems to have taken a pro-fat position, a line of thinking that I explore further in this book and is concerned with reducing the social stigmatisation of fat people. My guess is that this is why they read *The Obesity Epidemic* as endorsing the ideas that 'diets don't work' or that 'fat people aren't fat due to gluttony'. Actually, *The Obesity Epidemic* made no such arguments. Rather, it attempted to show something very different: finding definitive empirical proof for the effectiveness of diets or the comparatively high dietary intake of fat people was extremely difficult. In other words, this reviewer seems to have mistaken a book about the science of body weight for one about fat people. If nothing else, 'unbiased' was something Jan and I never claimed to be.

While the first reviewer seems to have missed our central arguments about science, the second reviewer (who identifies themselves as the Executive Director of the American Obesity Association) has over-read this dimension. Our caveats that we wanted to speak specifically about obesity science and not science in general have clearly fallen on deaf ears. Our point was not that all science is pointless. Rather, we argued that working out the physiological complexities of body weight at the level of the individual was all very well, but that this was a very separate matter to understanding the food and physical activity behaviours of millions of people in changing social, cultural, geographical and economic circumstances. In other words, the physiology of body weight is unlikely to shed any light on the emergence of something called an 'obesity epidemic'. And far from suggesting that people's thinking about body weight would never change – a most unlikely claim given our respective social science backgrounds – our criticism was specifically directed at those who claimed that changes in the science of body weight would *ipso facto* lead to more humane and rational ways of thinking amongst the general population. While scientific advances might in some cases contribute to a more just society, we made what I still think is the straightforward point that the relationship between knowledge and ethics was much more tenuous, unpredictable and even perverse. For example, then, as now, I do not see how new knowledge about human physiology or the genetics of body weight will make people less likely to see obesity as a personal moral failing.

Taken together, what I think these reactions to *The Obesity Epidemic* capture is the way people's moral and ideological predispositions shape the way they read, think and advocate when it comes to human body weight. In *The End of the Obesity Epidemic* my aim is to get inside the rhetoric of a wide range of obesity researchers, writers and commentators. In my view, this is one of the most important contributions an academic can make. That is, rather than converting the reader to a particular set of truths, my hope is to contribute to the reader's capacity to make their own critical and informed judgements about the truth of body weight.

Inevitably, there will be those who will dismiss my arguments here on the grounds that I see myself as ideologically pure or neutral. So, in addressing this issue, let me be as clear as I can about the position from which I will speak in this book.

First, I am an intellectual pragmatist, which, amongst other things, means I strive, however imperfectly, to see things from multiple points of view. While this may sound like a claim to neutrality, it is more a gesture towards an overriding scepticism towards alleged universal truths, be they scientific, religious, philosophical or any other kind. For me, intellectual pragmatism means that there is always another question to be asked and that, while the business of day-to-day living means having faith in a certain number of apparently reliable truths (such as the sun coming up in the morning and the wisdom of moving out of the path of oncoming buses), this is not a luxury that extends to the world of ideas. And although it is these days fashionable to deride the proponents of something called 'relativism', I believe that we live in a physical universe that is utterly indifferent to human concepts such as truth or god or beauty. This does not mean that I think truth, god or beauty are unimportant concepts, but rather that I take them to be concepts invented by people and imposed on the world in order to bring a measure of subjective order and coherence to our experience of it.

Second, however, I also assume that many readers will care little about my own personal convictions – a point that probably applies as equally to my general philosophical standpoint as it does to my views on obesity. This confers on the writer a certain freedom, I think, to be more free ranging and to offer the reader food for thought rather than definitive truth.

Third, I take it for granted that many of my own biases will be more obvious to others than to me, that others will see things that I am too myopic to see, but that this fact does not disqualify me (or anyone else) from speaking or attempting to critique received ways of thinking.

The end?

Much has changed since *The Obesity Epidemic* was published. For one thing, in both popular and academic spheres obesity rhetoric has grown, if anything, even more shrill. In some cases the predictions and lamentations of obesity experts have verged on the bizarre and it is partly these extremes that I consider in the next chapter. Over and above sheer rhetorical intensity, I also show how the obesity epidemic has spawned a number of what we might call 'rhetorical viruses'. For example, commentators of one sort or another have been prepared to predict that today's children will die younger than their parents. This prediction is made repeatedly in scientific journal articles, popular books, newspapers, television news bulletins and, in my experience, in polite conversation. In reality, only a very small number of studies have tackled the question of obesity's impact on life expectancy and these are mostly specific to the United States. Needless to say, this has not stopped the claim being made all over world with an unselfconscious solemnity that invites scrutiny. While it is at least theoretically possible, it seems unlikely to be something that will happen in all Western countries at the same time. My point here is that statements of this kind are not, in any straightforward sense, scientific. Rather, they are sound-bite viruses that have spread for no other reason than their sheer dramatic effect.

Is a rhetorical environment of this kind sustainable? Does there come a point when the penny must drop, when the words of experts and commentators become so unhinged from any empirical foundation that they lose even the superficial ring of science? Of course, these are hardly scientific questions themselves, but I do propose in Chapter 2 that obesity rhetoric increasingly over-reached itself in the first decade of the twenty-first century – a situation that probably helped to generate its own backlash of opposing points of view. Perhaps the emergence of opposing views was inevitable. However, by charting the heights (or depths) of obesity rhetoric I do want to suggest that hyperbole surely generates its own resistance and that this resistance represents an important turning point in the history of the obesity epidemic.

This leads to the first and most straightforward sense in which I will talk about the end of the obesity epidemic. In Chapter 3 I discuss evidence that obesity rates in many parts of the world have either slowed, plateaued or declined, in stark contrast to the claim that they are accelerating out of control. In some countries these trends appear to have begun over a decade ago.

It scarcely needs to be anticipated that this will not be a popular claim. Not for the last time then, I stress that an 'end' in this context does not mean that there are no longer any obese people or that there are uniform body weight trends in every region of the world. Rather, what *has* come to an end is the situation that is most obviously captured in the term 'epidemic' and the language of its proponents: the idea of a dangerously out-of-control situation. While the thirty years prior to 2000 were characterised by fairly generalised obesity rate increases across the Western world, this book argues that this is not the case any more, nor has it been so for about ten years. So, although my primary point of disagreement in previous research has concerned the health consequences of increasing obesity, *The End of the Obesity Epidemic* argues that the most credible component of the alarmists' case – unambiguously climbing obesity rates – is now also crumbling. The obesity epidemic is at an end because its core empirical claim is now untenable.

There will be those who will accuse me of splitting hairs. In particular, some obesity researchers concede that the rhetoric of 'crisis' and 'epidemic' may have been a little overblown, but add that the situation is still dire and, therefore, a little hyperbole is forgivable. But this qualification completely misses the arguments I made in *The Obesity Epidemic* and will develop in this book. In the past I have said that the situation is *much* less serious than the one described by the overwhelming majority of obesity researchers, a claim I develop in Chapter 4 by looking at recent official reports concerning the health of a number of Western countries. However, the new and, I think, more important argument presented in this book is that the medical and obesity research community has consistently misrepresented the trajectory of global obesity rates. On both counts – the seriousness of obesity and the trajectory of obesity rates – my divergence from the apparent view of mainstream obesity science is substantial. This is not a matter of splitting hairs.

Chapter 4 asks readers to look at the health of a small group of Western nations in the grip of an alleged obesity crisis. Although I have less space here than is needed to settle the matter, I try to at least pose a simple question: What happens to the obesity epidemic if we look at health not through the lens of obesity, but from a more global perspective? Is it just possible that obesity looks like a much more frightening problem only so long as obesity is the only thing one looks at? Or, to paraphrase Kipling, what do they know of obesity who only obesity know?

By the end of Chapter 4 I hope to have at least made a compelling case for questioning the idea of an ongoing and intractable obesity crisis. I hope also to have explained, in part, how the language of crisis started, spread and has the potential to mislead us. But rather than this just being a matter of semantics, in Chapter 5 my colleague Carolyn Vander Schee and I consider the way crisis rhetoric has led to social policies that have the potential to affect many of us, in both small and significant ways. Although any number of examples could be offered, we focus on the way schools and children have become the focus of anti-obesity policy in the United States. We think there are things to learn from this context, not just about the way misguided thinking leads to bad social policies, but also about the obesity epidemic itself. In fact, rather than the enactment of significant amounts of anti-obesity policy and legislation signalling the recognition of a real and present danger, we think it is actually a sign that the obesity epidemic is over.

By 2010, the window of opportunity for obesity experts to remake society according to their dreams had closed. Without them noticing, the obesity epidemic's numerical steam had begun to escape and the precious attention of politicians and policy-makers had begun to move on. The obesity epidemic had ended in two different but equally important ways: the first statistical and the second political.

The end of consensus

Before 2005 there was scarcely any such thing as a debate about the obesity epidemic per se. It is true that doctors, scientists and others had been arguing over the relative contribution of diet and physical inactivity to body weight for over a century and that, in more recent years, the role of genetics has attracted some interest. It is also true that the first edition of Glen Gaesser's book *Big Fat Lies* was published in 1996 and that, before this, the scientific literature had been lightly sprinkled with articles questioning the health consequences of overweight and obesity (for example, Ernsberger and Haskew 1987; Frank 1993; Kassirer and Angell 1998; Wooley and Garner 1991).

My point, though, is that prior to a moment somewhere around the middle of the current decade, the idea that dissenting views about the obesity epidemic existed could simply be ignored in the scientific literature and had not yet registered in the mass media. It is only quite recently that leading obesity researchers have begun to make grudging concessions towards obesity sceptics, such as the following from a *New England Journal of Medicine* editorial:

> Like global warming, the obesity epidemic is a looming crisis that requires action before all the scientific evidence is in. And as with climate change, some have questioned experts' forecasts, doubting the far-reaching impact of obesity, though scepticism is gradually being overcome by accumulating data.
>
> (Ludwig 2007: 2326)

No doubt the existence of sceptics is partly a reaction against the ubiquity and intensity of talk of an obesity epidemic – a case of an opposite, if not quite equal, reaction. However, surely Ludwig is also acknowledging here that, in contrast to the past, obesity sceptics were now far greater in number, publishing more books and articles and, to some extent, catching the media's attention. While Ludwig obviously has little patience for the arguments of sceptics, he can no longer act as if they do not exist.

The number of obesity sceptics has grown in recent years and they are the focus of Chapters 6 and 7. Taken together, these writers have generated a desperately needed counter-balance to the pervasive idea of an obesity crisis and, if nothing else, have offered readers alternative ways of thinking about the issue. However, it is common for obesity sceptics to be lumped together, especially by sceptics themselves, potentially giving the impression that they make the same arguments and reach similar conclusions. This is very far from the case.

These chapters have two distinct purposes. First, I try to show that the obesity epidemic's period of unchecked rhetorical dominance has ended. This, the third ending I describe in this book, is perhaps the most important of all since it potentially ushers in a period in which the objectives of obesity alarmists may need to be scaled down and their rhetoric modified in light of the criticisms that have been levelled against them. Of course, whether this happens will depend partly on the extent to which obesity sceptics are able to find a broad and influential audience for their views.

Readers of *The Obesity Epidemic* will be aware that Jan Wright and I were less concerned with converting readers to an alternative set of truths than we were with destabilising received ideas about obesity. Our message was that obesity science does not lend itself to zealous certainty and it is this, as opposed to some watertight new truth, that casts doubt on the idea that we are in the midst of a global health catastrophe. In other words, we argued that uncertainty was its own critique, sufficient in itself. This is a very different analysis from that offered by some other obesity sceptics, especially those discussed in Chapter 6, who explicitly describe themselves as the bastions of pure, unbiased truth. With telltale quote marks, I call this group of writers the 'empirical sceptics' not because I think their assessment of the scientific data is beyond question, but because this is how they represent themselves.

So, while I want to show that a vigorous opposition to obesity epidemic rhetoric exists, I do not want to suggest that this literature is without its own tensions. My interest in points of difference rather than consensus will become even more obvious as I turn in Chapter 7 to the work of obesity sceptics writing more from an academic social science or social activist perspective. While there are significant areas of overlap between the writers I survey in these two chapters, the social scientists are more inclined to start from an assumed truth about obesity than, as with the 'empirical sceptics', to conspicuously assert it. Rather than spending time assessing the science of obesity, these writers take it for granted that others have already demonstrated the errors and exaggerations of mainstream obesity science. They do this because they have a completely different agenda. For this group, whom I will call the 'ideological sceptics', the focus of analysis is oppression, although the nature and target of this oppression varies. For some, the obesity epidemic is an example of the oppression of women, while others see it as oppressing non-white people or children or the poor or the overweight and obese themselves. Once again, I need to stress that I do not call this group 'ideological sceptics' because they are more ideologically driven than any other group. The term is in one respect just a shorthand convenience that helps me to distinguish them from the 'empiricals'. However, given that this group does not dwell on the science of obesity and that they begin instead from the idea that obesity medicine and science are forms of oppression, the term 'ideological sceptics' does, I think, capture an important dimension of their work.

Over the course of Chapters 6 and 7 I hope to show that, taken together, obesity sceptics make an enormous range of divergent and plainly contradictory claims and arguments. This is important because it helps us to see that the obesity epidemic is not simply the clash of sceptics and alarmists. If there is a truth that I want to prosecute in these two chapters it is that understanding the obesity epidemic is not just or even a matter of deciding which is the side of truth and which the side of lies. The bad news for readers hoping to find a coherent set of ideas in the sceptics' camp is that the differences between sceptics are just as wide, if not wider, than the differences between sceptics and alarmists. I want to show that there are no easy alliances here, no comfortable synergies that will make it straightforward to work out where one stands. I want to show that coming to understandings about why the obesity epidemic happened, whether it matters and what we should do about it is a hugely complex undertaking that does not lend itself to the safety of pre-conceived certainties. And underlying all of this is my assertion that it is the slow burn of scientific uncertainty that undermines any claim to fully understand what is going on.

A number of points of clarification are necessary before going any further. Throughout this book I will talk about 'obesity researchers' and 'obesity experts'. For the most part I take these terms to be interchangeable. However, in some cases I have used 'obesity expert' to refer to a person who is speaking as a representative of an obesity-related organisation. In some cases these representatives are also researchers in their own right, but in other cases this was unclear. In any event, for the purposes of this book obesity researchers and obesity experts make up what I call the 'obesity research community', a term I use simply to group together all those who appear to talk about obesity with some degree of professional expertise.

On a perhaps slightly more contentious note, I will also use the terms 'obesity science' and 'obesity science and medicine'. For reasons that will become clearer in later chapters, I have intentionally avoided talking generally about 'science' or 'medicine' or even 'medical science'. In short though, this book is not about science or medicine per se and I have no interest in generalising about these large and diverse social institutions. The focus of this book is specifically the work of people who study obesity and treat obese people in a wide range of clinical settings. Besides, not all obesity research is medical. For instance, it is at least debatable whether we should think of epidemiologists, exercise scientists or public health researchers as 'medical researchers'. More clear-cut though, there are obesity researchers who study the built environment, law, public policy or even my own field of physical education. So, the term 'obesity science' attempts to capture the huge diversity of researchers and academics who study obesity. For a variety of reasons, I am also confident that at least some readers will object to calling all obesity research 'science'. Although this is a debate that interests me, the question of who does and does not deserve to be called a 'scientist' is one that I avoid in this book. For my purposes, 'obesity scientists' and 'obesity researchers' are the same people.

All of this is perhaps a long-winded way of saying that I am interested in the things that are written in research journals as well what obesity experts of various stripes say and write in other contexts, such as print and electronic media.

In *The Obesity Epidemic* I tended to place 'obesity epidemic' in quote marks. I have dispensed with this practice in this book purely to avoid typographical clutter. I am certainly no more inclined to use the term without qualification than in any of my previous work. The word 'obesity' itself is used mostly to mean the technical categories of 'overweight' (a Body Mass Index (BMI) of between 25.0 and 29.9) and 'obesity' (a BMI above 30.0) unless I have indicated otherwise. This is a slightly complex matter since when most people talk about the obesity epidemic they usually do so, often unwittingly, in a way that collapses these two categories, thereby greatly exaggerating the number of people who actually meet the technical definition of obesity. In fact, it is doubtful whether the idea of an obesity epidemic would exist at all without this conceptual slippage. Nonetheless, I have avoided using the term 'overweight and obesity', once again, for brevity's sake and have distinguished between the two when necessary. This book uses the word 'obesity' by itself because this is the word the world uses to talk about the body weight crisis that we are supposedly in.

Last, this book is about obesity in Western countries. I am aware of course that this is not an easily definable category. I considered using 'industrialised democracies' but decided it was an unnecessary mouthful. By 'Western', I am referring to those countries most conventionally grouped together as English-speaking democracies, such as the United States, Canada, Australia and the United Kingdom, as well as the countries of Western and northern Europe, such as France, Switzerland and Sweden. Generalisations are dangerous, but these are by and large the countries in which most obesity research has been carried out and which are most often mentioned by obesity researchers when they talk about the obesity epidemic. I understand that obesity is considered a serious matter in many other countries, but this book focuses on the countries where the obesity epidemic was first announced. At any rate, this is not particularly out of step with obesity science literature itself, which regularly refers to the obesity epidemic as the product of Western lifestyles.

This book's title refers to the 'end' of the obesity epidemic for three reasons. First, there is now consistent evidence that obesity rates are levelling off. In addition, the health of Western populations remains robust and life expectancy is rising. And while some obesity alarmists are beginning to walk away from their earlier mortality warnings and, as a result, shift their focus to morbidity, research data here also paint a complex and contradictory picture. Second, there is evidence that policy-makers have adopted a stance that attempts to give the impression of significant action against obesity while expending the least possible effort. In other words, those who sought to convince policy-makers of the need for an all-out co-ordinated war on obesity, harnessing all arms of government, have not succeeded. Instead, anti-obesity policy formation now sits vaguely in the middle of Western governments' 'to do' lists with little sign much is about to change. Third, the hyperbole of alarmist rhetoric has bred its own backlash so that as early as 2008 even a few politicians were prepared to openly question whether the obesity epidemic had been exaggerated – an unthinkable situation only a year or two previous.

2 Worse than global warming

In *The Obesity Epidemic* Jan Wright and I devoted a chapter to a comparison between the rhetoric of modern obesity science and that of the mass media. On the whole, we argued that there was actually little to choose between the hyperbolic language of both. While we might generally expect scientists to speak about their areas of expertise in a more sober, qualified and cautious manner than the media, in the world of the obesity epidemic no such distinction applies. We were able to find no claim about the looming obesity crisis, no matter how apocalyptic or far-fetched, that did not have its origins in the research literature or the published commentary of obesity scientists.

We made this comparison, first, because we wanted to show that the obesity epidemic was not simply being driven by a sensationalist or opportunistic media. In fact, unlike many other modern health panics, we found not a single example of an obesity scientist or expert complaining about being misrepresented in the media. As far as I am able to tell, this remains true in 2010.

Our second reason for focusing on the feverish pitch of obesity commentary, regardless of where it appeared, stemmed from our interest in the uses and effects of exaggeration. We argued that exaggeration matters because it is clear that Western media has fed upon the opinions and predictions of obesity scientists and that public discussion about obesity has largely been framed by their exaggerations. This discussion, in turn, has shaped the kinds of policies and actions that might be seen as reasonable, radical or based on evidence. So, while a certain policy might previously have seemed extreme or heavy handed, the same policy might begin to look more reasonable if the problem it purportedly addresses is regularly described as a 'crisis'.

This chapter is also about exaggeration, although I have been careful not to cover the same ground described in *The Obesity Epidemic* or duplicate the work of others. Rather, my purpose here is to set the scene for following chapters, but particularly Chapter 3, in which I consider recent research into overweight and obesity prevalence across the Western world. In this respect at least, this book follows a method I have used in virtually all of my obesity research, offering examples of alarmist rhetoric and then comparing these with published research.

There are, however, two other aspects of obesity rhetoric that I focus on here that, to my knowledge, have not been discussed in detail elsewhere.

First, I want to draw attention to the way a small number of specific rhetorical flourishes are endlessly recycled and, rather like viruses, passed from person to person, mutating but keeping their essential structure. Many writers have pointed out the flaws, mistakes and exaggerations of obesity science and the overheated language of the reporting mass media. Taking a slightly different tack, this chapter explores what we might call 'pure rhetoric', where the truth or otherwise of certain statements is not really the point. It is a world where language is used, more or less knowingly, not even with the intention of scientific simplification but as a tool in itself, floating free of science, in order to have an effect on readers and listeners.

Second, I want to show how these rhetorical viruses have become public property, untethered to temporal or geographical context. While a claim like 'America is the fattest country in the world' is repeatedly made, apparently without much consideration of its veracity, it is still a claim about a particular place and therefore, at least asserts an empirical fact about a specific part of the world. Likewise, the idea that obesity causes heart disease, while also contentious, is still grounded in a set of scientific propositions. The kind of statements I discuss in this chapter are, in a sense, universal. They belong to no one and everyone, nowhere and therefore everywhere. As we will see, they can be used in conjunction with virtually any other obesity-related claim and offered as a justification for virtually any course of action. Taken together, it is the promiscuity and universality of these rhetorical viruses – to say nothing of their sheer perversity – that demands particular critical attention. But first, a little background.

When too many deaths are barely enough

There was perhaps no other story about the obesity epidemic that so perfectly captured the nature of modern obesity science and its symbiotic relationship with the mass media. While the news that obesity kills 300,000 (and later 400,000) Americans every year was a perfectly formed and instantly repeatable sound-bite, it was also, depending on your point of view, either a ghastly or amusing exaggeration. Others (for example, Oliver 2006; Basham, Gori and Luik 2006) have charted the history of this statistic in more detail, but its basic trajectory is worth recounting briefly.

Although a small number of earlier studies are sometimes cited (particularly Amler and Eddins 1987 and McGinnis and Foege 1993), there seems to be general agreement that a 1999 paper in the *Journal of the American Medical Association* by Allison and colleagues (Allison, Fontaine, Manson, Stevens and VanItallie 1999) was the first attempt, in the context of increasing anxiety about population body weights, to estimate the number of American deaths attributable to obesity. The year is significant in that it coincides with the period in which the obesity epidemic as an idea appears to have been born. In fact, an argument could be made that Allison and colleagues' paper was one of the opening scientific salvos in the looming war on fatness. At around the same time the American Obesity Association organised a conference called 'Obesity: The Public Health Crisis'. Held on the 15th and 16th of September 1999, a press release announced that the 'conference brings, for the first time ever, this chronic disease into the public policy arena' (Riskworld.com 1999). Interestingly, the press release also highlights how the attention generated by the obesity epidemic around the years 1999 and 2000 was not based on startling new and conclusive scientific findings, but rather years of concerted advocacy by committed individuals: 'Founded in 1995, the American Obesity Association (AOA) is a non-profit organization whose fundamental mission is to have obesity regarded as a disease of epidemic proportions' (Riskworld.com 1999).

Allison and colleagues based their estimates on five large prospective cohort studies and, using 1991 as their year of analysis, asked: '. . . how many fewer would have died by the end of that year if all of the obese people alive at the beginning of the year had not been obese . . .?' (1999: 1530). Their conclusion was that obesity killed about 300,000 Americans every year, although they stress a number of times that this 'probably underestimates' (1537) the real figure. The paper was subsequently criticised on many grounds, but possibly most often because, as the authors themselves concede, '. . . our calculations assume that all (controlling for age, sex, and smoking) excess mortality in obese people is due to obesity' (1536). In other words, the paper's conclusions are based on the idea that if a person with a BMI above 25 dies, it must have been their fatness that killed them, no matter what the cause of death. Given that the paper set itself the task of estimating how many American deaths overweight and obesity caused, this assumption gives the paper an unmistakably self-fulfilling, circular quality since the answer is basically assumed in the question.

A great deal of the discussion about the statistic also concerned the significant financial links between the study's authors, the weight loss industry and, in particular, the pharmaceutical corporations developing and marketing weight loss drugs. There were those who argued that these links completely rendered existing mortality estimates untrustworthy, while others countered by pointing out that research sponsorship was simply the norm for all public health research conducted by the major American research institutions. Whether these arguments offer opposing explanations or, instead, are perfectly compatible descriptions of the same thing remains an open question today.

For my purposes here, though, the important point is that this study delivered to the world a simple round number that could now be circulated, repeated and, most important, easily grasped by journalists and their readers. It was a genie that once out of the bottle would prove impossible to control. It quickly became one of the most frequently quoted statistics in scientific history.

Allison and colleagues' estimate was followed in 2004 by 'Actual causes of death in the United States, 2000', a paper by researchers from the Centers for Disease Control and Prevention (CDC) that claimed that obesity killed not 300,000 Americans each year but 400,000 (Mokdad, Marks, Stroup and Gerberding 2004). The study was immediately engulfed in controversy not only for methodological reasons, but also because of reports of internal dissent, compromised quality controls and cover-up at the CDC. This led to a government investigation into the statistic, an internal review at the CDC and, most sensationally of all, a new study by other CDC researchers, using National Health and Nutrition Examination Survey data, that put the number of 'excess deaths' attributable to overweight and obesity (about 26,000) at a fraction of the earlier estimates (Flegal, Graubard, Williamson and Gail 2005). Controversially, the study found that overweight was associated with fewer non-cancer and non-cardiovascular disease deaths than 'normal' weight and was not associated with cancer or cardiovascular disease mortality at all (for examples of media reporting of the excess deaths controversy see Stein 2004 and Gibbs 2005).

This is not at all to suggest that Flegal and colleagues' estimates are beyond question. This kind of epidemiological research relies on a single measure of a person's BMI and, because of the large sample sizes involved, cannot account for weight changes during the period of time under investigation. This is a particular problem if one is inclined to accept the general observation that people tend to put on weight as they get older since it raises the possibility that a person could die 'obese' even though the study may have classified them as 'normal weight'.

In passing, the extent to which the proponents of '400,000 deaths' may have gone out on a scientific limb becomes apparent if we consider similar estimates in other countries. For example, in a study published in the *Canadian Journal of Public Health*, Katzmarzyk and Ardern (2004) calculated that overweight and obesity killed 4,321 Canadians each year and 57,181 between 1985 and 2000. The population of the United States, currently about 308 million, is a little less than ten times higher than that of Canada at about 33 million. It is true also that obesity prevalence is somewhat higher in the United States. But in very rough terms, Mokdad and colleagues' yearly death rate of 400,000 is about 100 times higher than Katzmarzyk and Ardern's Canadian estimate of just over 4000. Either obesity is about a ten-fold more deadly state in the United States than it is in Canada or, more likely, we are talking about a field of study unencumbered by agreed standards of method or analysis.

The methodological complexities generated by the excess deaths controversy are still a matter of debate today – not surprising given the high stakes. Involving two of the world's largest and most important health and medical research organisations, the CDC and the National Institutes of Health, the controversy attracted considerable media attention and threatened significant damage to the reputations of high-profile researchers and bureaucrats.

In his strident and curmudgeonly negative assessment of modern epidemiological science, John Brignell (2000) argues that simple statistical assertions about the health risk of anything should always arouse our suspicions. If we take at all seriously the idea that calculating health risk is an extremely messy and inexact science, then the glibness of round numbers are a clear warning that serious liberties may have been taken with the truth of the matter at hand. Writing before the obesity epidemic had lurched into full rhetorical stride, he cites the example of smoking:

> It is disturbingly frequent for the most blatant and gross falsehoods to be issued in press articles and broadcasts with no attempt at justification. A subject that will come up in this book with rather monotonous regularity is

smoking. One of the most repeated numbers from the anti smoking campaign is that it causes 400,000 premature deaths in the USA each year. This number is a total fabrication.

(Brignell 2000: 23)

My point here is not to cast doubt on the health risks of smoking or even to uncritically accept Brignell's assertion about the 'fabrication' of smoking-related mortality statistics. What I think is interesting is, first, the curious similarity between smoking and obesity mortality estimates and, second, the way big, round and highly contestable numbers are blithely deployed in public discussions of health. This is not to argue that smoking-related or obesity-related estimates about premature death are necessarily wrong; it is at least theoretically possible that one or other statistic corresponds to some hidden Platonic truth out there somewhere. Rather, in drawing attention to the enormous scientific uncertainty that is obscured by the assertion that fatness kills 400,000 Americans a year, my argument is that this statistic was never actually a statistic at all, at least not for very long. At a moment in history when a scientific community had, it seems, decided on a course of action designed to alarm and provoke, the idea of 300,000 or 400,000 deaths became an ideal rhetorical tool. Its scientific credentials became not so much debatable as inconsequential.

How big?

How big a problem is obesity? This is obviously a complex and probably unanswerable question. But as many public health advocates have argued, complexity and uncertainty are not much help when it comes to raising awareness and changing minds. It is important to remember also that although the obesity epidemic has been a global news story for about ten years, there are still obesity experts and commentators who think the problem is not being taken nearly seriously enough (for example, Stanton 2009; Swinburn 2008). They see this as happening on two levels. First, at the individual level, the argument goes that we have become so inured to the sight of obese people that we no longer recognise ourselves or our children as dangerously fat. Second, Western governments are blamed for being either too short-sighted or insufficiently brave to implement rigorous anti-obesity policies (for example, Delpeuch, Maire, Monnier and Holdsworth 2009). Western societies are, they argue, sleepwalking into a public health catastrophe.

It is not always clear what level of heightened vigilance would be enough for some obesity experts, but we can at least gain a sense of the urgency they feel by paying attention to the words they use.

Although they are quite rare, statistical comparisons of the public health challenges facing Western countries, even those intent on maximizing the threat of increasing body weights, tend to place obesity below smoking. That there is an issue to be debated is at least acknowledged by some authors. Writing in the journal *Diabetes, Obesity and Metabolism*, Peterbaugh (2009: 557) says of obesity: 'This arguably has become the greatest threat to the nation's present and future health'. Amongst the more outspoken and most-quoted obesity experts, however, even a small concession to uncertainty like this is rare.

For Paul Zimmet, who in 2008 was Director of the International Diabetes Institute, and Garry Jennings, Director of the Baker Heart Research Institute, the time for subtlety has clearly passed. In an article that appeared in the Australian newspaper *The Age*, these high-profile obesity experts warned:

> This new epidemic is our greatest public health concern and we need a popu-
> lation-based public health strategy to beat it . . . Obesity is the single most
> important challenge for public health in the 21st century. More than 1.5 bil-
> lion adults worldwide and 10% of children are now overweight or obese.
>
> (Zimmet and Jennings 2008)

Curiously, in the same article Zimmet and Jennings go on to say that 'This *may well be* the single most important challenge for public health in the 21st century' (2008, my emphasis), raising the question of whether they think obesity really is the world's greatest health challenge or simply a contender. This could, of course, simply be an editorial error. If not, it is, I think, a small taste of the way some obesity experts employ language. Rather than aiming for precision, one senses a kind of flailing about in order to press the right emotional button and create the desired sense of urgency. So, having said that obesity is 'our greatest public health concern' and then that it 'may well be the single most important challenge for public health', they then hit on another sound-bite to conclude the article: 'We don't have the luxury of time to deal with this epidemic – it's as big a threat as global warming and bird flu' (2008).

Were one of a mind to hold the authors strictly to the letter of their claims, obesity emerges simultaneously as more serious than bird flu, equally serious as bird flu and merely vying with bird flu for biggest threat status. This is to say nothing of the statement that seems bizarrely to equate the relative serious-ness of global warming, bird flu and obesity. Obviously, though, looking for this kind of coherence would be to over-analyse the words of these experts; the point being that for modern obesity science obesity can be whatever our speaker wants it to be.

While we might wonder whether (or hope?) there is a forgivable spur-of-the-moment quality to Zimmet and Jennings's comparisons with global warming and bird flu, it turns out that these are actually lines from a much-repeated script. Zimmet was one of the headline speakers at a large international obesity confer-ence held in Sydney in 2006. CBS News reported:

> The world is in the grip of a fat pandemic that threatens to overwhelm every
> country's health system with diseases such as diabetes and heart disease
> and shorten the life span of future generations, experts at an international
> conference warned on Sunday.
>
> 'Obesity is an international scourge,' Prof. Paul Zimmet, the chairman of
> the meeting of more than 2,500 experts and health officials, told delegates

in a speech opening the International Congress on Obesity. 'This insidious, creeping pandemic of obesity is now engulfing the entire world.'

'It's as big a threat as global warming and bird flu,' said Zimmet, an Australian expert on diabetes.

(2006)

Equating obesity with the threat of climate change has become commonplace. In 2007, BBC Online reported that 'The Health Secretary Alan Johnson recently said obesity was a problem "on the scale of climate change"' (Murphy 2007). This echoed the warning of the British government sponsored Foresight Report, *Tackling Obesities – Future Projects*, that the British obesity problem was 'as bad as climate risk' (Foresight 2005). And as we saw in the previous chapter, endocrinologist and outspoken Harvard Medical School academic David Ludwig has written in the *New England Journal of Medicine* that, 'Like global warming, the obesity epidemic is a looming crisis that requires action before all the scientific evidence is in' (2007: 2326).

Once again at the risk of over-analysis, it is worth dwelling for a moment on the idea that the obesity epidemic is as serious a problem as global warming. Perhaps the most startling thing about this claim is that, to the best of my knowledge, nobody actually knows how serious a problem global warming is. More to the point, it is not clear what obesity experts who make this claim know about global warming. Many readers will be aware that even the most gloomy climate scientists accept that predictions about the planet's future climate are subject to a wide margin of error. What, then, are obesity scientists actually saying when they compare obesity to global warming?

Some readers may think this an uncharitable question. Perhaps a more reasonable interpretation of the claim that rising obesity levels are as serious as global warming is that it is not so much a scientific claim, but rather a metaphoric one. In this interpretation, the person who makes the claim is trying to say that both global warming and the obesity epidemic are extremely serious phenomena that deserve urgent action. And yet, if this second interpretation is correct, we must turn back to the scientific evidence, something I will do in Chapters 3 and 4. In short, the obesity = global warming proposition does not simply say that rising obesity levels will lead to an increase in some diseases and have a moderate effect on the amount of premature death. Rather, this claims says that obesity is the kind of problem that requires policy-makers to prioritise it above all others and will lead to catastrophic, irreparable and long-term damage to our way of life. As Paul Zimmett puts it, obesity is 'engulfing the world'.

Global warming and bird flu have not by any means been the only points of comparison. Speaking to a US audience, the former director of the CDC, Julie L. Gerberding, is reported to have claimed that 'If you looked at any epidemic – whether it's influenza or plague from the Middle Ages – they are not as serious as the epidemic of obesity in terms of the health impact on our country and our society' (Kvicala 2003). In an article for the *Boston Globe*, David Ludwig and another prominent obesity researcher, Kelly Brownell, wrote that 'The obesity epidemic threatens the foundations of our society as would a massive SARS outbreak' (Ludwig and Brownell: A13).

Whatever else we might say about these kinds of predictions and comparisons, it is clear that they circulate and reproduce themselves, sometimes slightly mutated, but similar enough to be sure that they stem from the same core sentiment. And as I have already argued, it is striking how similar the rhetoric of experts and non-experts is. Take, for example, the following from the website of Australian politician Guy Barnett: 'Obesity and diabetes are now recognised as the worst health epidemics in world history, with 100,000 more Australians contracting diabetes and 200,000 becoming obese each year' (Barnett 2006). It is tempting to wonder to whom the author was referring when they wrote this obvious hyperbole about 'world history' and asserted that it was 'now recognised'. We might even dismiss this as the over-heated language of a politician trying to attract attention. But if pressed, Mr Barnett could have pointed to claims made by organisations like the American Obesity Association. Its president, Richard Atkinson, is responsible for a series of sound-bites, such as 'Medicine has never seen an epidemic of this proportion' (Food Online 2000). Another, that obesity is 'the most prevalent, fatal, chronic disease of the 21st century', is attributed to Atkinson and Morgan Downey, also of the American Obesity Association (American Obesity Association 2005) and recycled regularly in print and online media.

While apparently first made by Atkinson in 1999, almost exactly the same statement – 'Obesity is the most prevalent, fatal, chronic, relapsing disorder of the 21st century' – sits, without attribution of any kind, on the website of the Washington D.C. based Obesity Society ten years later (The Obesity Society 2009). In fact, these are the first words the reader encounters on the Society's 'What is obesity' page. In passing, as an academic I react with suspicion to the lack of a citation for this claim and recall the advice I give students to always try to support their arguments with supporting evidence. However, one wonders whether in contexts like this, where academic niceties matter less, a citation might actually draw the attention of a reader to the need for evidence and, therefore, the potential contestability of the claim being made. Made without reference to evidence, it is possible that this kind of crude rhetorical sweep is rendered more, not less, credible to the average reader by virtue of its apparently seamless certainty.

In defending his website's claim about obesity and world history, Mr Barnett might also refer to the writing of Mike Adams, whom the website DiabetesAnswers. org describes as the 'Author of over twelve books, and fifteen hundred articles on natural health', as well as being 'considered the most prolific writer on natural health today' (DiabetesAnswers.org 2004). For Adams, the scourge of obesity has turned Americans into not only 'the most diseased people on the planet' but also 'the most diseased group of people in the history of human civilization' (Adams 2004). Once these kinds of statements are made and circulate in Western culture, the possibility for any other claim, no matter how dubious, to be seen as rank hysteria is surely diminished.

Speaking at the 2009 American Psychological Association's conference, epidemiologist Steven Blair is reported to have told delegates that physical activity is 'the biggest public health problem of the 21st century' (ScienceDaily 2009). This is interesting for a couple of reasons, not least because Blair has been a leading advocate for the 'fat, fit and healthy' hypothesis – the idea that how fit and physically active a person is matters much more than how much they weigh (for more discussion of Blair's research see Chapter 6). But if the report is accurate, Blair's prediction is also as puzzling and meaningless as those quoted above about obesity. A huge amount of uncertainty surrounds the exact health benefits of physical activity, not least because the health benefits of physical activity may turn out to vary from person to person. Perhaps what we are seeing here is another example of the way advocates for particular positions apparently decide that the only way to attract the attention of public policy-makers is through wild hyperbole.

More generally, it is also striking how this kind of prediction, be it about physical activity, obesity or anything else, appears to see a uniformly serious situation in all parts of the Western world. This is highly improbable given that, in the case of obesity, rates differ from country to country and there is general agreement that excess body fat affects different ethnic groups in different ways. In other words, there would seem to be an obvious prima facie case against sweeping universal claims about the present and predictions about the future.

How bad?

When new buzzwords and phrases appear it is often impossible to know when or by whom they were first used. However, by 2010 there could surely have been few Westerners who had not at least heard that obesity would kill today's children at an earlier age than their parents. The recycling of this phrase seems to have happened in a similar fashion to the claims about obesity-related deaths I discussed above. However, there is at least one interesting difference between these two rhetorical viruses.

The idea of children dying en masse younger than their parents does not appear even to owe its origins to a published research paper, flawed or otherwise. Instead, it is sometimes traced to Texas Children's Hospital's William Klish, who is quoted in a 2002 edition of the *Houston Chronicle* (Ackerman 2002). There is no clear indication that Klish meant to imply that this was a claim based on science or even that it was particularly likely. What we can say is that the idea caught on. Immediately after predicting that one-third of all children born in the United States in the year 2000 would develop Type II diabetes, the country's Surgeon General Richard Carmona told a 2004 Senate sub-committee that: 'Because of the increasing rates of obesity, unhealthy eating habits, and physical inactivity, we may see the first generation that will be less healthy and have a shorter life expectancy than their parents' (United States Department of Health and Human Services 2004).

In one form or another, the prediction of an obesity-led decline in life expectancy was made by a string of American obesity experts and public office holders up to and including Bill Clinton. Launching the Clinton Foundation's 'Alliance for a

Healthier Generation' initiative, the former president warned: 'For the first time in American history, our current generation of children could live shorter lives than their parents' (Clinton Foundation 2005).

In time, a scholarly attempt was made to substantiate this claim. Olshansky and colleagues' article 'A potential decline in life expectancy in the United States in the 21st century' appeared in a March 2005 edition of The *New England Journal of Medicine*. The authors wrote:

> An informed approach to forecasting life expectancy should rely on trends in health and mortality that may be observed in the current population. Forecasting life expectancy by extrapolating from the past is like forecasting the weather on the basis of its history. Looking out the window, we see a threatening storm – obesity – that will, if unchecked, have a negative effect on life expectancy. Despite widespread knowledge about how to reduce the severity of the problem, observed trends in obesity continue to worsen. These trends threaten to diminish the health and life expectancy of current and future generations.
>
> (Olshansky et al. 2005: 1138)

These opening lines from the article's abstract at least acknowledge the hazards attached to making predictions, especially in light of obesity science's well-known knowledge gaps. But with this caveat out of the way, the authors move to what 'will' happen and the 'threats' that await us:

> Our conservative estimate is that life expectancy at birth in the United States would be higher by 0.33 to 0.93 year for white males, 0.30 to 0.81 year for white females, 0.30 to 1.08 years for black males, and 0.21 to 0.73 year for black females if obesity did not exist. Assuming that current rates of death associated with obesity remain constant in this century, the overall negative effect of obesity on life expectancy in the United States is a reduction in life expectancy of one third to three fourths of a year. This reduction in life expectancy is not trivial – it is larger than the negative effect of all accidental deaths combined (e.g., accidents, homicide, and suicide), and there is reason to believe that it will rapidly approach and could exceed the negative effect that ischemic heart disease or cancer has on life expectancy.
>
> (Olshansky et al. 2005: 1140–1141)

Whether conservative or not, these are quickly superseded by more pessimistic predictions:

> These trends suggest that the relative influence of obesity on the life expectancy of future generations could be markedly worse than it is for current generations. In other words, the life-shortening effect of obesity could rise from its current level of about one third to three fourths of a year to two to five years, or more, in the coming decades, as the obese who are now at younger ages carry their elevated risk of death into middle and older ages.
>
> (Olshansky et al. 2005: 1141)

In the context of this article the proposition that obesity might lead to a decline in life expectancy of five years or more is made almost as a speculative throw-away line towards the end of the paper. It is not a claim that is based on detailed statistical analysis.

In the few years since its publication this single paper has accrued close to 1,000 citations for two main reasons. There is, of course, the obvious value of its apparently scientific findings to those wanting to emphasise the seriousness of the obesity epidemic. However, the paper has also been extensively criticised on a number of methodological grounds, two of which may be obvious to readers from the passages quoted above. First, the paper's predictions rest on a comparison with a world where no obesity at all exists. So even when the authors predict only a fraction of a life expectancy year lost to obesity, this is not based on a comparison between now and a United States that existed ten, twenty or thirty years ago. The comparison is with a United States that, as far as we know, has never existed.

Alert readers will have noticed also that Olshansky and colleagues base their calculations on the assumption that 'current rates of death associated with obesity remain constant in this century'. It is now widely recognised that this is not a robust assumption. For one thing, medical advances, such as new surgical procedures and drug therapies, mean that people who suffer from conditions that are statistically associated with obesity are less likely to die because of their illness. For another, there is consistent evidence that for any given BMI, today's obese Westerner tends to have a significantly better profile on risks factors such as blood pressure and cholesterol than his or her counterpart of a generation ago (McCarron, Davey Smith and Okasha 2002; Bennett et al. 2006; Ford et al. 2007). While there may be debate about how unhealthy a BMI above 30 actually is, there is some agreement that it is less unhealthy than it used to be.

There is a long list of other objections that have been raised against Olshansky and colleagues' calculations, including the obvious and serious charge of conceptual slippage. For example, if obesity causes heart disease and several common types of cancer, as many obesity researchers claim, how do you measure the discrete death tolls of obesity and heart disease and cancer? What sense does it make to talk of obesity-related deaths overtaking heart disease deaths if many – but not all – of the people killed by heart disease are also obese? It is perhaps more instructive to keep in mind that the authors of this paper include some of the most vocal advocates for classifying obesity as a discrete disease. In other words, just asking the question 'How many deaths does obesity cause?' indicates a pre-existing commitment to a contentious idea that obesity is itself a disease and not simply a risk factor for other diseases.

The confidence of Olshansky and colleagues in their findings does not appear to have been dented by widespread criticism. David Ludwig, one of the paper's co-authors, has been unrelenting in his warnings about the looming obesity crisis: 'My colleagues and I have predicted that pediatric obesity may shorten life expectancy in the United States by 2 to 5 years by midcentury – an effect equal to that of all cancers combined' (Ludwig 2007: 2325).

Elsewhere, other American researchers repeat this assertion without any reference to the objections that have been raised. Writing in *The Milbank Quarterly*, Adler and Stewart predict: 'Among other things, the diminishing rates of smoking have helped increase longevity, but the obesity epidemic may slow or even reverse the trend toward longer life expectancy' (2009: 50).

One of the things that has struck me about the constant recycling of this idea is the way it has acquired a kind public ownership. For example, the claim that today's children will live 'sicker and shorter lives than their parents' has become a kind of accidental cliché, whereby virtually anyone who needs to say something about obesity apparently feels free to claim it for themselves. Writing on behalf of America's National School Boards Association, Perkins and Piñeyro announce:

> This alarming rise holds true across the board for white, black, and Hispanic children, and numerous studies have shown that overweight children are more likely to experience serious health problems as adults. What that prognosis means is that this generation of children may be the first in our nation's history to live sicker and shorter lives than their parents.
>
> (2009: 32)

Notice the way the authors of this passage obscure the source of the analysis they offer. When they write 'What that prognosis means is that . . .', they imply that the prediction that follows comes from their own assessment of the evidence. At the very least, why 'that prognosis' means anything at all is not explained; it is simply delivered with an air of scientific seriousness. Having read dozens of passages of this kind over the last decade, my sense is that they offer us a glimpse of the alchemy that the obesity epidemic performs. In other words, this passage is a living, breathing example of an idea in the process of transformation from speculative after-thought into scientific fact.

Is it pedantry to reiterate here that Olshansky and colleagues' original paper calculated an obesity-driven decline in life expectancy of less than a year for most people and that their more gloomy predictions were, at best, guesses? In all the reincarnations of the United States life expectancy sound-bite I have never seen the actual statistics from Olshansky and colleagues' paper reproduced. Is this because a decline of between 0.33 to 0.93 of a year for white males and 0.30 to 0.81 for white females is not sufficiently attention grabbing? Whatever else is true about the longevity of future American generations, what this examples shows is that, in the here and now, the worse the news, the better it travels.

And travel is has. Writing recently in the *Canadian Medical Association Journal*, Harris, Kuramoto, Schulzer and Retallack (2009) lament obesity levels amongst Canadian young people and then note similar trends around the world. Remarkably, though, they then generalise about the health effect of 'these trends' in a way that leaves the reader little choice but to assume they mean that childhood obesity will have the same effect everywhere. Finally, citing Olshanskey and colleagues, they claim: 'This in turn may result in the first-ever decline in life expectancy in the developed world' (Harris, Kuramoto, Schulzer and Retallack 2009: 719). Do they mean in Canada? The entire developed world? Although the paper they cite to support this claim is based exclusively on American data, the authors do not even mention the United States and there is no sign that they have any qualms generalising from these data to their own or anybody else's country. In fact, Harris and colleagues provide us with a glorious example of the life expectancy sound-bite sprouting wings and landing very far from home.

As early as 2004 the American speculations of William Klish and Richard Carmona turned up in a United Kingdom House of Commons Health Select Committee on Obesity. Without the support of any systematic local life expectancy analysis, the report concluded that 'this will be the first generation where children die before their parents as a consequence of childhood obesity' (quoted in Evans 2006: 262).

In fact, as elsewhere, in the United Kingdom the life expectancy sound-bite quickly became a kind of default lens through which all obesity-related research could be interpreted. So when local experts were asked for a comment, it was always on hand. The 2006 release of National Health Survey statistics for 2004 on childhood obesity unleashed a storm of media coverage in which obesity experts like Colin Waine, Chairman of the England's National Obesity Forum, were quoted repeatedly:

> It really augurs very badly for the future health of the population as these children move from adolescence to adulthood. We are in danger of raising a generation of people who have a shorter life expectancy than their parents.
> (Carvel 2006: 1–2)

As early as 2004, Australian newspaper columnists like family values advocate Miranda Divine predicted that Australian children were headed for a 'ridiculously premature death' (2004: 15). Likewise, the life expectancy sound-bite has been eagerly received and deployed in New Zealand. In December 2003, New Zealand journalists and obesity experts were combining to predict not only declining life expectancy, but the extinction of New Zealand's indigenous Māori people:

> Obesity is expected to result in a shortened life expectancy for New Zealanders. Wayne Cutfield, director of endocrinology at Auckland Starship Children's Hospital, says there will be a drop in life expectancy 'very soon'. 'In time, obesity will shorten life expectancy – in less than 20 years,' Professor Cutfield says . . . Norman Sharpe, medical director of the Heart Foundation, agrees that obesity will cause a drop in life expectancy. 'In Britain they are now predicting for the first time that children growing up today will have a shorter life expectancy than their parents because of the obesity problem and New Zealand is almost certainly in the same situation,' Professor Sharpe says.
> (Fox 2003)

Although we cannot be sure who penned the words, a New Zealand government website had former Prime Minister Helen Clark adding her voice to the chorus:

Unless something changes the current generation of New Zealand children may very well be the first to die at a younger age than their parents . . . This issue is potentially the greatest single threat to the health of New Zealand families, and our biggest public health challenge.

(Clark 2006 quoted in Burrows 2009: 129)

Where did Helen Clark or her advisors get this idea from? Judging by some of these quotations, it is at least possible that it was picked up by someone in the New Zealand government who had heard it from a New Zealand obesity expert who had, in turn, borrowed it from obesity commentators in the United Kingdom who, as we have seen, picked it up from the United States. Writing in the *New Zealand Medical Journal*, Grant and Bassin uncritically regurgitate Mrs Clark's phrase:

When launching *Mission On*, Prime Minister Helen Clark said there is a need to improve nutrition intake and reverse the declining levels of physical activity. It was suggested that unless something changes in our living environment and the way we approach the modern lifestyle, it is possible the current generation of young New Zealanders may be the first generation to die younger than their parents.

(Grant and Bassin 2007: 2)

The sheer ubiquity of this idea in obesity rhetoric makes it a difficult phenomenon to generalise about. However, my sense is that over time people who repeat the decline in life expectancy claim have done so with an increasing air of certainty. In their recent book *Globesity: A Planet Out of Control?*, a group of European researchers wrote:

To sum up: the more you are overweight, the sooner you die. The optimum size, for anyone who aspires to live to be a hundred, can be expressed as a BMI score of between 18 and 25. It seems probable that life expectancy, which has steadily risen in the developed world, may soon become shorter as a result of obesity. Unless we can overcome this epidemic, today's young people may well have unhealthier and shorter lives than their parents enjoyed before them.

(Delpeuch, Maire, Monnier and Holdsworth 2009: 29)

The indiscriminate sweep of this passage is remarkable and the authors make no effort to specify who 'we' or 'today's children' are.

At the end of 2009, the *New England Journal of Medicine* published a new study that attempted to predict the effect of rising obesity on the life expectancy of Americans. The researchers' conclusion was that the life expectancy of an eighteen-year-old would rise by 3.76 years by 2020, but that obesity will slow this increase by 0.71 years (Stewart, Cutler and Rosen 2009). It is possibly inevitable that the life expectancy of some Westerners must plateau and perhaps even decline at some point in the future. The idea that it will be obesity that brings about this change anywhere in the Western world, though, is very far from certain.

The idea of declining life expectancies in Western countries continues to be trapped in a kind of echo chamber, its reverberations now an indecipherable cacophony. Journalists quote experts who quote other experts and other journalists and so on in an unstoppable feedback loop. There are probably many reasons why this happens, but one is worth dwelling on for a moment. In an article for the *Journal of Public Policy* called 'Translating research into public policy', Harold Goldstein draws on his own work at the California Center for Public Health Advocacy to offer readers a step-by-step guide to mobilising policy-makers in the war on obesity. For Goldstein, the first two steps are to 'define a problem and describe it locally' and then to 'develop an effective policy solution' (Goldstein 2009: S18). However, the third step is perhaps the most instructive. Goldstein suggests researchers 'develop a convincing message' which includes crafting sound-bite reductions of research for maximum effect. Goldstein writes:

> Much of the political process is about communication. Toward that end, we work closely with a public relations firm to frame our messages – and the research on which they are based – and to develop convincing ways to tell our story.
> Here, for example, was our message about school food.
>
> - The problem: 'Childhood obesity rates have skyrocketed and schools are a part of the problem – they have become soda and junk food superstores.'
> - The effect: 'This could be the first generation of children in modern history to have a shorter life expectancy than their parents.'
> - The policy solution: 'It is time to get schools out of the junk food business.'
>
> (2009: S18)

Apparently, Goldstein thinks this is an example of developing what he calls a 'convincing message'. The point to take from this example, I think, is that when people who write about obesity talk of a convincing message, what they really have in mind is an alarming message. 'Convincing' in this context does not mean 'credible', but rather something that is likely to cause fear and, therefore, action.

While Goldstein may call this 'translating' research into public policy, what I see is closer to fairground magic. Goldstein's trick is to juxtapose three essentially unrelated statements: 'skyrocketing' obesity rates, the sale of junk food in American schools and declining life expectancies. Then, without giving the reader time to think, he moves on to a final and equally unrelated sound-bite. In fact, far from research being translated into public policy, there is no research here at all, just a series of rhetorical flourishes. And it is here that we see the magic performed by an idea like children dying younger than their parents. After all, in Goldstein's formulation virtually any obesity 'research' finding could have preceded it and any policy recommendation could have followed it. There are no rules; like the distracting wave of the magician's hand, any idea can be made to fit with any other idea so long as the reader can be diverted and dazzled by the spectre of death.

How many?

In his book about a year spent travelling to the strangest cultural festivals he could find, Australian writer Brian Thacker found himself at an Elvis Presley convention. He noted wryly, 'I once read that Elvis impersonators are growing at such a rate that, by the year 2050, the entire population of the planet will be Elvis impersonators' (Thacker 2004: 10). Amongst other things, Thacker was reflecting on the way this kind of prediction appeared regularly in the media to warn of some unpleasant social or medical trend.

It is hard to know how these predictions should be viewed. Providing the upward trend really is occurring, whatever it happens to be, it stands to reason that if it continues to happen it will one day affect everyone or be everywhere. On the other hand, since when has the rate of change of any real world phenomenon been strictly uniform from start to finish, extending indefinitely into the future?

With this in mind, there are some grounds for puzzlement about the regularity and seriousness with which predictions about the proportion of people who will be obese at some point in the future seem to be made. As with the previous sound-bites discussed in this chapter, only a small amount of systematic modelling designed to generate this kind of prediction has ever been carried out. Unlike, say, economics or meteorology, obesity is not a field of study that can call on elaborate technical procedures to make at least arguably educated forecasts about the future. For example, the field has no generally agreed upon theories or models that explain the reason for obesity rate changes. At the very least, the fact that many obesity researchers readily concede that we really do not know what has caused changes in the past should give one pause to wonder about the efficacy of any prediction concerning future obesity rates.

It is perhaps partly because of the lack of an underlying theoretical model that apparently serious obesity commentators like Paul Zimmet could feel sufficiently free to announce 'Obesity is an international scourge . . . This insidious, creeping pandemic of obesity is now engulfing the entire world' (CBS News 2006). In other words, without an agreed upon system for generating or evaluating predictions, obesity experts like Zimmet may actually be free to say whatever they want. And once said, this kind of prediction – if this is what it really is – is liable to be mimicked not just by journalists, but by other researchers. Delpeuch, Maire, Monnier and Holdsworth warn that 'we are beginning to realize that no society is immune from this plague, which is rapidly engulfing the whole of the globe' (2009: xv).

Scientific consideration is no guarantee of consensus, of course, but it is interesting to speculate whether its absence contributes to the wide range of predictions about future obesity prevalence that are made. In a 2007 article for the *Nursing Standard*, Tasmin Snow draws on one set of statistical predictions in order to urge British nurses to take a pro-active role in solving the obesity epidemic and thereby save the National Health Service from ruin:

> . . . latest estimates predict that by 2010, around 33 percent of men and 28 per cent of women will be obese. Obesity among children is also projected to rise, with the number of obese boys rising from 750,000 in 2003 to nearly 800,000

in 2010. The largest increases are expected among girls, with a 6 per cent rise in obesity rates expected between 2003 and 2010, by which time some 910,000 are expected to be obese. This equates to more than one fifth of those aged between two and 15.

(2007: 12)

Sky News (2009) has reported recently that 'experts' expect 'two thirds of all children will be overweight or obese by 2050'. Also in the United Kingdom but drawing on very different forecasts, journalist Helen Rumbelow writes with startling certainty for *Times Online* about a moment still forty years in the future:

> Now we all know that exercise is the best way to lose weight, in the same way that we all know that our obesity epidemic is a result of Western sloths sitting on our ever fatter bottoms. It's why chubby will be the new norm, with 90 per cent of today's children predicted to be overweight or obese adults by 2050, costing UK taxpayers £50 billion.
>
> (Rumbelow 2009)

This appears to be basically the same prediction as that attributed to British politician Alan Johnson:

> . . . health secretary Alan Johnson warned that nine out of 10 adults will be obese or overweight by 2050, and as the Government launches its most extensive drive to stem the growing epidemic by encouraging people to eat more healthily and take regular exercise.
>
> (Devlin 2008)

However, this is somewhat different from Johnson's own government report that:

> Our extrapolations indicate that on current trends, by 2015, 36% of males and 28% of females will be obese. By 2025, 47% and 36% respectively are estimated to be obese, and by 2050 the proportion of the population that is obese will be 60% of males and 50% of females.
>
> (McPherson, Marsh and Brown 2007: 13)

This is again slightly tweaked by the obesity researcher Susan Jebb in the magazine *Business Voice*: 'In the government's Foresight report on tackling obesity, we extrapolated current trends to reveal that 40 per cent of people could be obese by 2025, and 60 per cent by 2050' (2009: 50). In fact, given that many of the predictions about obesity in the United Kingdom come from the same source (the Foresight Report), it is remarkable how many authors offer different versions of what the report says. Take the following from the *Journal of Internal Medicine*: 'Increasing obesity rates are guaranteed under current circumstances: by 2050 60% of men and 40% of women will be clinically obese at a very conservative cost of £45.5 billion year' (James 2008: 347).

Estimates concerning the United States are equally idiosyncratic. As early as 1997 at least one leading obesity researcher was predicting that 100% of Americans would be obese by 2230 (Foreyt 1997). While an early and particularly bizarre case, this is an instructive example of the way some obesity experts have used prevalence forecasts. While the idea of obesity prevalence reaching 100% 230 years in the future feels, at least to me, a reassuringly long way away, the projection exists perhaps in the hope that its sheer cheek will be submerged under its potential to shock. It is, in other words, more sci-fi than science. Amazingly, it was to go on being cited uncritically in journals such as the *Journal of the Royal Society for the Promotion of Health* (Walker 2003) and *Nutrition in Clinical Practice* (Breen and Ireton-Jones 2004).

As unlikely as it might seem, the idea of 100% obesity prevalence does pop up in the media statements of obesity experts from time to time. Judith Stern of the American Obesity Association is often attributed with the following remark: 'If we don't try something new, in about 10 years everyone in the country will be overweight or obese' (Marini 2004: 1c).

Based on the dubious assumption (see Chapter 3) that American overweight and obesity rates are still going up and will continue to do so, Wang and Beydoun propose the following in the journal *Epidemiologic Reviews*:

> Currently, 66% of adults are overweight or obese; 16% of children and adolescents are overweight and 34% are at risk of overweight. Minority and low-socioeconomic-status groups are disproportionately affected at all ages. Annual increases in prevalence ranged from 0.3 to 0.9 percentage points across groups. By 2015, 75% of adults will be overweight or obese, and 41% will be obese.
>
> (2007: 6)

In an article titled 'Will All Americans Become Overweight or Obese?', the same authors extrapolate further in the journal *Obesity*:

> If these trends continue, by 2030, 86.3% adults will be overweight or obese; and 51.1%, obese. Black women (96.9%) and Mexican-American men (91.1%) would be the most affected. By 2048, all American adults would become overweight or obese, while black women will reach that state by 2034.
>
> (Wang, Beydoun, Liang, Caballero and Kumanyika 2008: 2323)

Compare these confident assessments to Baum's radically different calculations in the *Journal of Population Economics*. Here, the author attempts to predict future American obesity rates by taking into consideration expected changes in the country's racial make-up: 'These figures show that projected racial/ethnic composition changes initially increase the prevalence of obesity from 2005 to 2014 but decrease obesity thereafter, with an overall decrease from 29.79% in 2005 to 29.62% in 2050' (Baum 2007: 694).

One aspect likely to confuse readers is that some predictions are made about future obesity percentages and others concern only overweight, while still others combine the two. For example, what sense might a reader make of the statement 'Research indicates that if childhood obesity rates continue to soar, half of all Australian children will be overweight by the year 2025' (Masters 2007), found in an online news story? Does the author *really* mean that current 'obesity' rates have been used to calculate future rates of 'overweight'? Or is this simply a mistaken mixing of terms? Likewise, the following gloomy passage appeared in an article for a 2001 edition of Australian *Marie Claire* magazine. It is interesting to wonder how many readers would have picked up on the distinction between the passage's prediction about overweight, but the article's overall focus on Australian rates of obesity:

> Dr David Crawford, National Heart Foundation Nutrition Research fellow at Deakin University, has been researching the epidemic of obesity for the past 10 years. 'Epidemic is not too strong a word,' he insists. 'Being overweight is affecting all people, all strata of society. By 2025, nearly every Australian adult will be overweight.'
>
> (Johnson 2001: 234)

From a presumably more reliable source than *Marie Claire* – a report by two Australian academics to the Australian Preventative Health Taskforce – we read:

> The prevalence of overweight and obesity in Australia has been increasing steadily over the past 30 years. According to the National Preventative Health Taskforce's discussion paper: *Australia the healthiest country by 2020*, it has been estimated that if current trends continue unabated over the next 20 years, nearly three-quarters of the Australian population will be overweight or obese in 2025.
>
> (Gray and Holman 2009: 3)

Gloomier still is the Australian state of Victoria's Department of Human Services (2008), which expects 83.2% of Australian men over the age of twenty and 74.6% of women to be overweight or obese by 2025.

Perhaps the most significant aspect of obesity forecasts, whether in the media or academic journals, is that they are not based on any theoretical model or rationale. Forecasters never attempt to construct an explanation of past trends that then feeds into predictions about the future. As I have said, this is partly because obesity experts have no theory about the past apart from a set of sweeping generalisations about 'modern lifestyles', generalisations that are mathematically inert. Future social trends are rarely factored in so that, for obesity experts, the future must always be nothing more than a pale imitation of an arbitrarily chosen moment in the past. This is much more folk superstition than it is science.

What this means, of course, is that any vaguely plausible prediction is as good as any other. As a result, obesity experts rarely, if ever, chastise each other for the rashness of each other's predictions. Instead, they have simply referenced, quoted and echoed each other to the point that obesity forecasts are now not so much scientific claims as background noise.

Predictions about the future are a fact of life and as many obesity forecasters say, generating knowledge about the future makes planning for it at least a theoretically more precise exercise. And yet, I must admit to being bewildered by the variety of obesity predictions that are made and, even more so, the conviction with which they are sometimes delivered. Whether or not readers are inclined to put credence in them, their existence is less important than the realization that, with a very few notable exceptions, these predictions rest on the idea of an increasing or, at best, unchanging and presumably never-ending rate of increase. This is precisely the supposition that underpins the astonishingly bold prediction, published in the *International Journal of Obesity*, that by 2030 57.8% of the world's population, or 3.3 billion people, will be overweight or obese (Kelly, Yang, Chen, Reynolds and He 2008). And it is also this logic that drives the authors of the book *Globesity: A Planet Out of Control* to ask in apparent seriousness: 'Is the whole world fated to become obese? Are we to look forward to societies in which everyone, give or take the odd exception, will be overweight?' (Delpeuch, Maire, Monnier and Holdsworth 2009: 159).

There is, it seems, no end in sight. Or, as Gary Mason put it in Canada's *Globe and Mail* newspaper much more succinctly than I: 'In the meantime we'll just keep getting bigger and bigger and bigger and bigger' (2005: A13).

How fast?

One of the least-discussed difficulties associated with predicting future rates of obesity is that there is actually no agreement about how quickly obesity rates are changing. In the case of forecasts about whole countries or the world, the fact that different parts of the world are changing at different rates (Lobstein, Baur and Uauy 2004) must be ignored in order to make predictions about the whole. In addition, the real rate of change for any population would depend on a long list of variables, including what definition of 'obesity' is used, the time period over which previous rates of change are calculated and, particularly important, the population's age profile.

These complexities aside, predictions based on the assumption of steady future rates of change apparently disregard assertions within the obesity research community that obesity rates are increasing at increasing rate. While I am aware of only a few obesity forecasts that have factored in increasing rates of change, it is a claim that has been regularly made.

Reporting on research into obesity rates amongst English children up to the year 1998, Lobstein, James and Cole (2003: 1136) reported an 'accelerating trend' and that 'There is a clear and urgent need for policies to be introduced to ensure that the *present* trends are halted and reversed' (1137, my emphasis). The idea of 'present trends' in this article is interesting because it refers to data that, by the time of the article's publication, were five years old. A couple of years later Stamatakis,

Primatesta, Chinn, Rona and Falascheti (2005: 1002) conducted a follow-up analysis of 2003 data and concluded that 'These results showed that the upward trends in overweight and obesity in children noted by other authors over the 1990s are continuing into the 2000s and, more alarmingly, that the rate of increase has accelerated over the last decade' (2005: 1002).

Generalising about European children, Jackson-Leach and Lobstein have written as recently as 2006 that 'Overweight and obesity prevalence in children is increasing. Furthermore, the significant linear trends in the annualised increments indicate that the rate of change is itself increasing: i.e., prevalence rates are not rising at a constant rate but are accelerating' (2006: 29).

In Australia, the practice of making pronouncements about the present based on old data is equally widespread. Booth and colleagues have reported in the *American Journal of Clinical Nutrition* that 'The prevalence of overweight and obesity [amongst Australian children] is not only increasing, it is accelerating' (2003: 35). Also in 2003, Booth was quoted in the media saying 'The prevalence of overweight and obesity is not only increasing, it is accelerating' (Teutsch 2003: 25). Similar to the Lobstein example above, Booth's claim relates to research into Australian childhood obesity between the years 1985 and 1997. In other words, Booth makes a claim about something that is going on now – 'obesity is not only increasing, it is accelerating' – when, his data concerns a period of time some six years in the past. On one level this is understandable given the complexity of this kind of research and the length of time it sometimes takes for results to be published. However, no caveats, such as the theoretical possibility that obesity rates might have slowed or reversed in the intervening years, were reported and I am not aware of any being offered elsewhere.

Writing more recently in the *International Journal of Pediatric Obesity*, Norton, Dollman, Martin and Harten are, if anything, more strident about the present and more alarmed about what they take to be current rates of change:

> The prevalence rate for overweight and obesity among children in Australia continues to climb and we predict it will approach adult rates within the next 30 years. [. . .] The increasing rate of overweight children in Australia, shown in Figure 2, is astounding. The data indicate overweight prevalence was relatively stable for much of the last century but accelerated in the early 1970s and continues to gain momentum.
>
> (2006: 232, 237)

More recent still is Peterbaugh's assessment of American obesity, in *Diabetes, Obesity and Metabolism*, that: 'Americans are more obese than ever, and the rates of obesity seem to be accelerating' (2009: 557).

It is interesting that as early as 2000 journalists were reporting the possibility of exponential rises in obesity rates, especially for children. From American *Newsweek* magazine:

> If the trend has continued – and many experts believe it has *accelerated* – one child in three is now either overweight or at risk of becoming so. No race

or class has been spared, and many youngsters are already suffering health consequences.

(Cowley 2000: 43, emphasis in original)

In 2005 Philip James, Chair of the International Obesity Task Force, is reported to have told a European Union obesity conference: 'It [obesity] took off in the 1980s and looks as if it was accelerating in the last five to 10 years . . . It's beginning to look as if we have an exponential rise' (Smith 2005). As with other obesity sound-bites, this is the kind of statement that could be, and in fact was, picked up and recycled in the media (for example, see also American Health Network 2005).

While it has been common practice over the last ten years for articles in research journals to talk about 'rampant obesity' (Raghuwanshi, Kirschner, Xenachis, Ediale and Amir 2001: 346) or 'burgeoning obesity' (Bonfiglioli, King, Smith, Chapman and Holding 2007: 58), there is actually very little evidence that obesity prevalence in Western countries was increasing more quickly after the year 2000 than before it. And yet, over the last ten years Western media have fed off the statements of experts to paint a picture of a situation careering out of control. Newspaper headlines continued to announce an 'obesity explosion' in the United States (Rumbach 2006) and Britain (Alexander 2008) deep into the new century's first decade. Even the Australian Prime Minister was prepared to use the term 'obesity explosion' in late 2009 on talkback radio to describe the situation in his own country (Prime Minister of Australia 2009). It is hard to think of a more precise illustration of the way the obesity epidemic has turned itself into widely understood sound-bites and, in this case, one that captures the sense of a rapidly worsening situation.

In one sense, the idea of rapidly increasing rates of obesity is actually what the obesity epidemic *is*. Without it, obesity has the potential to settle back into the medical scenery from whence it came. But like the other obesity sound-bites discussed in this chapter, it is not in any straightforward or, actually, important sense a scientific idea. Because obesity rates were very low in Western countries up until the beginning of the 1970s, any significant increase after this point was always going to look proportionally large. In this context, it was also possible that rates of increase might change from one survey to the next – a situation that could easily have existed without then drawing the conclusion that the situation was exploding exponentially. In fact, with hindsight we can see that right from the beginning of the obesity epidemic the situation was being described as 'explosive' and little has changed in the intervening ten years. It is an idea that has passed into common usage, deployed by people across the globe in a way that assumes that the listener or reader knows exactly what is meant.

In the following chapters I will offer reasons to doubt many of the commonly circulating ideas about the extent and seriousness of the obesity epidemic in Western countries. For the moment, though, I want to emphasise that each of the four viral sound-bites described above has been sustained by scarcely a whiff of scientific evidence. From so little, so much has grown. And while they appear to say a great deal, even gentle probing shows that each is an empty rhetorical shell, saying almost nothing and designed not to make a scientific case, but to create the impression of one.

Although I have made the point already, it is crucial to emphasise that my portrait of obesity rhetoric is not a whimsical exercise seeking simply to poke fun at people whose views I do not share. The stakes are much higher than this. My argument here it is that these sound-bites are the very substance of the obesity epidemic. They are what transforms obesity from a run-of-the-mill public health problem into a 'crisis' and what licenses its advocates to call for far-reaching, expensive and radical public health responses and policies. In other words, finishing where I began this chapter, the crime that is alleged in this and Chapters 3, 4 and 5 is one of gross, widespread, continuous exaggeration.

At the risk of confusing matters, my focus on exaggeration is important for another reason. In Chapters 6 and 7 I turn to the work of other obesity sceptics who, in their various ways, also want to dispute the claims of obesity science. As we will see, obesity science is accused of a great many sins besides mere exaggeration by its various sceptics. So, while the issue of exaggeration is what motivates my criticisms, it also signals a point of separation between the positions taken by other sceptics and myself.

This discussion, however, is for later. For now, we turn to the pivotal issue of obesity prevalence around the Western world.

3   The inconvenience of good news

Although body weight is a complex scientific matter, at a public policy level there is probably only one point that matters: how many overweight and obese people are there? After all, continuing improvements in the general health of Western populations does not seem to have been enough to convince Western policy-makers that the obesity dragon has been slain or that it is less fierce than first thought. Faced with calls for drastic action from a wide range of lobby groups, Western governments have simply been unable to say 'What crisis?'

Rather, it has been the sheer number of people classified as overweight and obese that has carried the day. Oliver (2006), for example, argues that, beginning in 1998, the worldwide circulation of a set of PowerPoint slides pictorially representing rising levels of overweight and obesity across the United States was a hugely effective and influential intervention by obesity scientists determined to bring about urgent policy action. So, when media reports have announced that, say, 60% of a nation's population is overweight or obese, this has been a sufficiently shocking statistic, coupled crucially with endless repetition, to precipitate action. Put another way, it seems telling that Western politicians have tended not to stake their determination to do something about obesity on the parlous state of their nation's health. Attacking the government's inaction, a Scottish Conservative Party health spokesperson described the figures for childhood obesity, not children themselves, as 'appalling' (English 2005). Likewise, in 2008 the Australian Health Minister Nicola Roxon said that obesity statistics, not Australians, were 'staggering' (Rodgers 2008).

This may seem an unimportant distinction. However, focusing on numbers rather than people allows the speaker to sound less like a scolding parent admonishing children for their bad behaviour. Similarly, talking about statistics rather than health means that the general improvements in Western health, for which governments normally try to take credit, can be sidestepped.

From my perspective, though, reducing the number of people classified as obese is not the same thing as reducing the number of people who, for example, die from cancer. Fewer cancer deaths mean more people alive than otherwise would have been dead, whereas it is not at all clear what fewer people classified as overweight or obese would actually mean for a nation's health. As I show in Chapter 4, rising fatness around the world in recent decades has not coincided with declining health. This does not mean that rising levels of overweight and obesity will have no effect on health. However, it does underscore the point that it is hard to know what effect, if any, small or even large drops in overweight and obesity would have. It is this uncertainty that makes the public policy focus on overweight and obesity statistics per se a notable and, in my view, perverse development.

With the rhetorical landscape discussed in Chapter 2 as our backdrop, I now want to review published research that casts doubt on the picture of rampant obesity in all parts of the Western world. The question I want to raise here is a simple one: to what extent have the combined forces of obesity science, amplified through the media, misrepresented the seriousness of the Western world's obesity problem?

North America

Reading popular and academic articles about the obesity epidemic in the United States means being constantly confronted with matter-of-fact and yet utterly conflicting statements. While it is true that many obesity experts continue to speak and write about 'exploding' rates of obesity, there has been a small amount of discussion about apparently hopeful signs in the National Health and Nutrition Examination Survey data. In 2006, under the headline 'Obesity rates among American women falling', the *Medical News Today* website reported:

> While more and more children and adult males are becoming obese in the USA, rates for women seem to be falling. 33.2% of American women were obese in 2004, a slight drop from 33.4% in 2000. This is the first bit of encouraging news regarding the ever-increasing weight of Americans in general over the last twenty years. Healthcare professionals in the USA say this offers a glimmer of hope. If women adopt healthier lifestyles, this could eventually be passed on to other members of the family. Unfortunately, men and children are putting on the weight faster than women are losing it.
>
> (Nordqvist 2006)

Even in 2006, the statement that American men and children were 'putting on the weight faster than women are losing it' was questionable. As we will see, there is some evidence that obesity rates among men did not change after 2004 and were not, as *Medical News Today* implies, galloping out of control. And yet, a reader of this article in 2006 might in 2008 have come across 'Obesity epidemic seen slowing but not falling' on the website *BNET*:

> 'Obesity has been increasing in prevalence over the last several decade [sic]. But we are starting to see a leveling off among women, and it doesn't look like we've seen any major increases among children and teens over the last several years,' said Karen Hunter, a spokeswoman for the Centers for Disease Control and Prevention. 'But it's not decreasing, either.'
>
> A study published in May in the Journal of the American Medical Association found that between 1999 and 2006, overweight and obesity among children in

the United States stayed stable at about 32 percent. By contrast, between 1980 and 2004, the percentage of children ages 6 to 11 who were obese increased from 6.5 percent to 18.8 percent; among those ages 12 to 19, the rate increased from 5 percent in 1980 to 17.4 percent in 2004.

(*BNET* 2008)

The reader of these two articles is left with an obvious question: Were American childhood overweight and obesity rates going up after 1999 or not?

Perhaps the most significant empirical counterpoint to the narrative of increasing obesity in the United States appeared in 2007. For some years, a group of researchers located at the National Center for Health Statistics (NCHS), a division of the United States' Centers for Disease Control and Prevention (CDC), have been reporting on the body weights of Americans using data from the CDC's National Health and Nutrition Examination Survey (NHANES). While not by any means the only research group to monitor American body weights, their oversight of the large NHANES data set makes theirs an extremely significant, if not dominant, voice.

In a 2007 publication concerning obesity in American adults, the researchers reported:

> Among men, the prevalence was 31.1% in 2003–2004 and 33.3% in 2005–2006. There was no statistically significant change. Among women, the prevalence in 2003–2004 was 33.2% and in 2005–2006 it was 35.3%. Again, these estimates were not statistically different from each other.
>
> (Ogden, Carroll, McDowell and Flegal 2007: 1)

Let us now compare this analysis with the accompanying graph, presented below in Figure 3.1. These data throw up a series of points of interest. If we take the obesity statistics for women alone, we might wonder whether the graph does not actually show that obesity prevalence has been stable for a longer period of time than the 2003–2004 and 2005–2006 interval reported here. An earlier paper by the CDC researchers (Ogden et al. 2006) supplies the data points for the graph. They reported that in 1999–2000 the obesity prevalence for American women twenty years or older was 33.4%, 33.3% in 2001–2002 and 33.2% in the 2003–2004 survey. It is worth reiterating that the 2007 report that announced 'no change' between 2003–2004 and 2005–2006 was based on a statistically non-significant rise from 33.2% to 35.3%. This non-significant rise is actually the first rise of any kind, statistically significant or otherwise, since 1999–2000. In fact, based on these numbers, the change between 2003–2004 and 2005–2006 is actually bigger than the change between 1999–2000 and 2005–2006. Any way we look at these data there appear to have been no significant changes in the obesity rates of American women, taken as an undifferentiated group, at least since the beginning of the twenty-first century.

For American men the picture is slightly different. The data points are 27.5% in 1999–2000, 27.8% in 2001–2002 and 31.1% in 2003–2004. The rise from 1999–2000 to 2005–2006 comes in at what seems a not insubstantial 5.8% (27.5% to

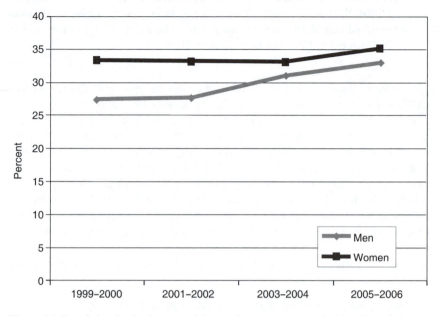

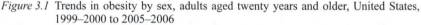

Figure 3.1 Trends in obesity by sex, adults aged twenty years and older, United States, 1999–2000 to 2005–2006

Source: Adapted from Ogden et al. (2007)

33.3%), at least compared to women. One possible interpretation of these data, therefore, is that increasing obesity prevalence amongst American men has slowed or stopped, although this happened later than for women. It is also interesting that the gap between men and women's obesity appears to be small and converging on zero. This finding is in direct contrast with years of obesity researchers warning about the particular problem of obesity amongst girls and women.

In early 2010, the CDC researchers published NHANES overweight and obesity rates for 2007–2008. These data confirmed the results of the 2005–2006 survey:

> For women, the prevalence of obesity showed no statistically significant changes over the 10-year period from 1999 through 2008. For men, there was a significant linear trend over the same period, but estimates for the period 2003–2004, 2005–2006, and 2007–2008 did not differ significantly from each other. These data suggest that the increases in the prevalence of obesity previously observed between 1976–1980 and 1988–1994, and between 1988–1994 and 1999–2003 may not be continuing at a similar level over the period 1999–2008, particularly for women but possibly for men.
>
> (Flegal, Carroll, Ogden and Curtin 2010: 240)

To say the very least, the contrast between these findings, suggesting a largely stable situation, and the general tone of obesity rhetoric in the United States over the last ten years is stark.

Returning to United States children, a 2008 paper published by CDC researchers in the *Journal of the American Medical Association*, also using NHANES data, found that 'The prevalence of high BMI for age among children and adolescents showed no significant changes between 2003–2004 and 2005–2006' (Ogden, Carroll and Flegal 2008: 2401). The researchers used three different definitions of 'high BMI': above the eighty-fifth, ninety-fifth and ninety-seventh percentile on standard BMI-for-age growth charts. Taken together, these cut-off points can be interpreted as covering what would otherwise be called 'childhood overweight and obesity'. Sample sizes of about 4,000 children were used for both 2003–2004 and 2005–2006 and included children from across the major ethnic groupings. The study compared data from four NHANES survey periods and concluded: 'No statistically significant trend in high BMI for age was found over the time periods 1999–2000, 2001–2002, 2003–2004, and 2005–2006' (Ogden, Carroll and Flegal 2008: 2404). Although there are differing absolute rates of overweight and obesity in different groups, the finding of no significant change in each BMI category was consistent for boys and girls and across ethnic groupings. And while in Chapter 2 we saw predictions in various countries of childhood overweight and obesity hitting 50% and higher, these data have overweight and obesity combined (above the eighty-fifth percentile) for American children between two and nineteen years of age at 31.9% and obesity (above the ninety-fifth percentile) at 11.3%.

As with the data for adults, the 2007–2008 NHANES survey has confirmed these earlier findings (Ogden, Carroll, Curtin, Lamb and Flegal 2010). Once again looking at three different measures of 'high BMI', the CDC researchers found that the only category that showed a statistically significant upward trend between 1999 and 2008 was boys above the ninety-seventh, a percentile finding that suggests that while almost all children have not become heavier, the number of very heavy boys has increased. The authors report:

> No statistically significant linear trends in high weight for recumbent length or high BMI were found over the time periods 1999–2000, 2001–2002, 2003–2004, 2005–2006, and 2007–2008 among girls and boys except among the very heaviest 6- through 19-year-old boys.
>
> (Ogden et al. 2010: 242)

This study also reported that the combined prevalence of overweight and obesity for American youth in 2007–2008 was 31.7%, a very far cry from the 46% by 2010 predicted by Youfa Wang (Johns Hopkins School of Public Health 2006), perhaps the most regularly cited forecasters in this area of study.

As well as reporting on the NHANES, the CDC also conducts what it calls the Pediatric Nutrition Surveillance System (PedNSS). Childhood obesity data from this scheme was most recently published in 'Obesity Prevalence Among Low-Income, Preschool-Aged Children: United States, 1998–2008' (Sharma et al. 2009). The report describes PedNSS as 'a state-based surveillance system that monitors the nutritional status of children from birth through age 4 years enrolled in federally funded programs that serve low-income children' (Sharma et al. 2009: 769). In each of the three years discussed in this report, 1998, 2003 and 2008, approximately 2 million low-income children aged two to four years were surveyed:

> The findings indicated that obesity prevalence among low-income, preschool-aged children increased steadily from 12.4% in 1998 to 14.5% in 2003, but subsequently remained essentially the same, with a 14.6% prevalence in 2008 ... Obesity increased across all racial/ethnic groups during 1998–2003, with the exception of Asian/Pacific Islander children. However, during 2003–2008, obesity remained stable among all groups except American Indian/Alaska Native children.
>
> (Sharma et al. 2009: 769)

Despite the existence of internationally accepted cut-off points, designating obesity in children as young as two remains a dubious empirical exercise. Nobody in obesity science knows the precise level at which childhood body fat begins to harm the health of a child or the adult they will become. Notwithstanding these limitations, the graph (see Figure 3.2) accompanying the PedNSS data suggests a couple of somewhat surprising trends, including the apparent leveling-off of obesity amongst low-income Hispanic and black children.

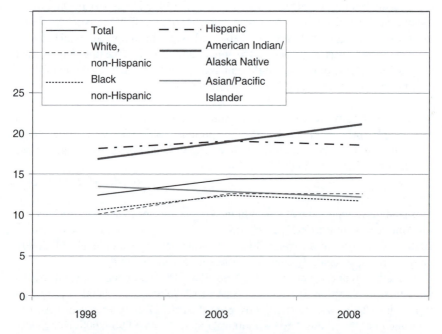

Figure 3.2 Change in obesity prevalence during 1998–2003 and 2003–2008 among children aged two to four years, by race/ethnicity

Source: PedNSS U.S. 1998–2008. Adapted from Sharma et al. (2009)

These results quite closely match those of the Youth Risk Behavior Surveillance System (YRBSS), another national health-related data collection scheme. The YRBSS collects data from children in both public and private schools in all fifty American states. Looking at trend data since 1999, the YRBSS has reported that 10.7% of children were obese in 1999, 10.5% in 2001, 12.1% in 2003, 13.1% in 2005 and 13.0% in 2007. YRBSS documents report no change in childhood obesity between 2005 and 2007, but the figure for 2003, 12.1%, has a 95% confidence range of between 10.8% and 13.6%, which raises the possibility of at least a slowing trend between 2003 and 2005 (YRBSS 2009).

One final and highly instructive example concerning obesity in the US is worth considering. 'The timing of the rise in U.S. obesity varies with measures of fatness' appeared recently in the journal *Economics and Human Biology* (Burkhauser, Cawley and Schmeiser 2009). For readers interested in the way obesity researchers sometimes ignore or fail to notice apparently important findings in their own data, this is an especially revealing case (see below for examples from Canada and Scotland).

The paper considered data from existing NHANES surveys (1971–2006) as well its predecessor, the National Health Examination Survey (1966–1970). According to the researchers, it is generally thought that obesity prevalence in the United States was stable through the 1960s and early 1970s and only began to rise sharply from the mid-1970s onwards. In other words, the standard view is that the obesity epidemic began with a bang about thirty-five years ago. In order to test this assumption, obesity prevalence measured by BMI for adults and youths aged twelve to seventeen years was compared with obesity prevalence measured by skinfold thickness, often considered by obesity researchers to be a more direct and therefore more reliable measure of fatness than the BMI. The researchers found that if we take skinfolds rather than BMI as our measure, obesity prevalence for adults and youth began to rise earlier and more gradually, at least from the mid-1960s and perhaps as early as the 1950s.

The authors of the paper make much of this finding. This is perfectly understandable since it was precisely the effect of comparing fatness measures that they originally sought to study. However, the paper concludes that this finding is important because it will help us to respond to the current obesity crisis. Is this justified? The researchers suggest that if we had used skinfold measurements rather than the BMI then we might have seen the obesity epidemic coming sooner and therefore taken action earlier. This is debatable on a number of levels not least because the levels at which skinfold measurements become an unambiguous health risk is not well understood. However, if we do as the authors suggest and shift our focus from the 1960s to the last ten years, the paper's data actually hint at a series of interesting conclusions that are mostly absent from its text.

First, while BMI obesity prevalence for US youth aged twelve to seventeen years in 2006 was 32.3%, the skinfold prevalence was 26.2%. In other words, the more direct measurement reduces childhood obesity by about 20%. For adults, the situation is completely the reverse. In 2006 aggregated adult BMI obesity prevalence was 31.8% and 43.4% when measured by skinfold thickness. This

discrepancy is caused by the much higher obesity prevalences for women produced by skinfold measurements compared to the BMI. To my eyes, this finding
suggests a number of misgivings about the entire enterprise of overweight and
obesity classification. While some readers might seize upon the higher skinfold
measurements as conclusive proof of an obesity crisis, I would reply by asking
whether the thresholds for skinfold obesity are simply too low. After all, there has
been very little study of the relationship between skinfold thickness – as opposed
to the BMI – and health; this point should cause us to pause before calling any
skinfold measurement 'obesity'. And while the authors of the paper do not say it,
for me there is an obvious question: does anybody really know what obesity as a
stable scientific entity is?

Closer to the focus of this chapter, though, almost without exception the paper's
graphs suggest that obesity, however measured, began to plateau and in some
cases decline in the 1990s, a point that draws no comment from the authors
whatsoever. A string of examples could be offered here. Aggregated data for boys
and girls shows that skinfold obesity reached 27.7% in the 1999–2000 survey,
has bounced up and down since that time and was 26.2% in 2005–2006. White
girls recorded a skinfold obesity prevalence of 20.1% in the 1988–1994 survey. A
number of surveys and more than a decade later in 2005–2006 this was virtually
unchanged at 20.6%. For black boys, BMI obesity was 37.3% in 1999–2000 and
29.2% in 2005–2006. For skinfold obesity the corresponding drop was from 28.4%
to 20.9%. For all male youths combined the change over the same time period
for skinfold obesity was 28.9% to 29.6%. A similar picture for adults emerges,
although the plateauing appears a little later, is more pronounced for women than
for men and is non-existent for black males.

Let me be clear. My point here is not to argue in favour of either the BMI
or skinfold thickness as a measurement of fatness. Obesity researchers are well
aware that different measurement techniques produce different numbers. What I
think is worth drawing attention to is the way this complex data set, which in many
ways counters received wisdom about American obesity, is simply glossed by the
paper's authors as confirming the upward spiral of obesity. To my eyes, the data
presented do nothing of the kind.

Let us pause for a moment before moving to other countries. Some readers
will be inclined to dismiss evidence of a levelling-out of obesity prevalence in
the United States and argue that, regardless of this trend, obesity is still too high.
My argument is that, on the contrary, whether or not obesity prevalences are too
high or not depends very much on their rate of change. Why? Because, as I will
show later in this book, there is some agreement that Western countries like the
United States are currently enjoying better overall health than at any time in their
history. This is a point I have made many times in print, the electronic media
and public debates without ever being challenged. Furthermore, at no stage have
I suggested that obesity is a completely insignificant heath issue now. Rather,
the core of my argument is that the obesity epidemic has been sold to the world
not on the state of our health today, for to do so would invite obvious questions
about how good general health could exist alongside unprecedented levels of

obesity. Rather, the obesity epidemic rests on warnings about the future – a future in which more and more people are expected to be unacceptably fat. Thoroughly alarmed American academics Finkelstein and Zuckerman capture the meaning of the obesity epidemic this way:

> Where will our soldiers and sailors and airmen come from? Where will our policemen and firemen come from if the youngsters today are on a trajectory that says they will be obese, laden with cardiovascular disease, increased cancers and a host of other diseases when they reach adulthood?
>
> (2008: 155)

But what if a different, less dramatic, more business-as-usual future awaits us? What then?

For the United States's northern neighbour, Canada, there is not much about obesity prevalence that can be said with a high level of confidence. Trying to develop a longitudinal picture is difficult since statistics for the last decade are a mixture of self-reported and objective measurements. Overall, though, available data suggest that obesity prevalence is considerably lower than in the United States.

Commentary on Canadian data also offers a reminder of how, when people are determined to tell a particular kind of story, they will see what they want to see. Take *The Obesity Epidemic in Canada*, a report produced by that country's Parliamentary Information and Research Service. The report begins its section on obesity prevalence by claiming that:

> Regardless of the specific studies or surveys used, the statistics are consistent in showing increasing rates of overweight and obesity in Canadian society over time. Between 1970–1972 and 1998, the proportion of Canadian adults considered overweight or obese increased from 40.0% to 50.7%. Figures 1A and 1B depict the results of a series of seven surveys conducted between 1970 and 1998, which show an increase in the share of Canadian men and women, respectively, who are considered overweight and obese.
>
> (Starky 2005: 3)

If we pause for a moment to gather the picture painted by these words in our minds, my guess is that at least some readers are seeing a steady increase in obesity prevalence across the near thirty-year period described, peaking in 1998 with no end in sight. And yet, the report's Figure 1A referred to here (Figure 3.3) presents a rather more complex picture.

Most people working in obesity research understand the perils of trying to read trends from one study to the next. Small differences in data collection and statistical procedures can render comparisons essentially meaningless. This is particularly true in the current example since many of the data are self-reported. However, on the surface at least, combined overweight and obesity for Canadian women appears to have decreased from the mid-1980s till the mid-1990s and then

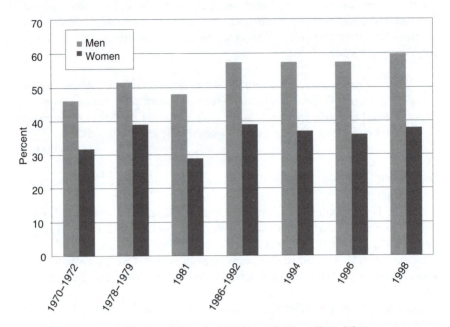

Figure 3.3 Prevalence of overweight including obesity for Canadian adults

Source: Adapted from Starky (2005)

risen slightly in the 1998 study. In fact, overweight and obesity prevalence looks essentially unchanged in the twenty years from 1978 to 1998, with the only significant jumps in the early 1970s and early 1980s. For men, there appears to have been only a very slight increase from 1986 to 1998. I submit to readers that this graph corroborates its accompanying text, quoted above, in only the most superficial way. Take also Figure 3.4, which presents prevalence rates for obesity alone.

Here, obesity amongst Canadian women appears to have peaked in the 1986–1992 survey and remained below that level at least until 1998. And while the upward trend for adult males appears to be unambiguously different, the increase from 1986–1992 to 1998 is still only three or four percentage points. Let me emphasise that I make no claim about the real prevalence of overweight and obesity amongst Canadian adults during the 1970s, 1980s and 1990s. As with all the studies and statistics discussed in this chapter, my purpose is to ask the reader whether these data match the picture of the explosive obesity crisis in Western countries that we have been warned about.

Later in *The Obesity Epidemic in Canada*, the document claims that combined adult overweight and obesity climbed from 48.5% in 2003 to 58.8% in 2004. For obesity alone the jump was from 15.4% to 23.4%. However, the document readily concedes that this jump is almost certainly an artifact of the transition from self-report to measured heights and weights.

Once again, although a mix of parent-reported and measured data, the

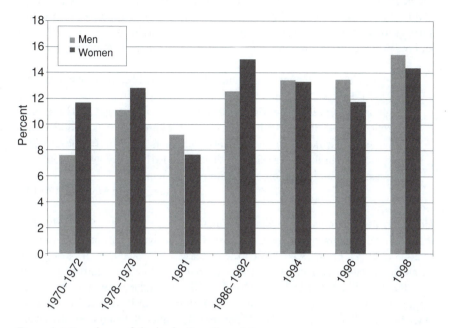

Figure 3.4 Prevalence of obesity for Canadian adults

Source: Adapted from Starky (2005)

document's account of childhood overweight and obesity in Canada cuts against the rhetoric of constant increase. For boys, it claims that overweight (excluding obesity) prevalence was 10.6% in 1981, rising to 32.6% in 1995–1996, and then falling to 29% in 2000–2001. For girls the corresponding rates are 13.1%, 26.6% and 27%. For boys' obesity, the percentages are 2.0%, 10.2% and 9% and 1.7%, 8.9% and 10% for girls. The report notes that 'According to one methodology, rates of overweight (including obesity) among children ages 7 to 13 increased by 200%–300% between 1981 and 2001, though they appear to have stabilised somewhat in recent years' (Starky 2005: 5).

The document then goes on to claim that overweight (excluding obesity) for boys and girls combined, using measured heights and weights, was 18.1% in 2004. This is well below the overweight prevalence reported for 1995–1996 (32.6% for boys and 26.6% for girls) that used parent-reported data that, as researchers constantly point out, tends to underestimate the real level of overweight and obesity. For obesity alone, the 2004 prevalence is 8.2%, once again below the parent-reported 1995–1996 scores (10.2% for boys and 8.9% for girls). Taken together, if these data have any validity at all, they suggest not that childhood obesity in Canada has 'stabilised in recent years', but rather that it stabilised a full decade before the publication date of *The Obesity Epidemic in Canada*.

Returning to adult obesity, another example of selective seeing appears in 'Prevalence of class I, II and III obesity in Canada', a short report in the *Canadian*

Medical Association Journal by leading obesity researcher Peter T. Katzmarzyk and Caitlin Mason (2006). The study combines data from a number of previous surveys to chart the trajectory of Canadian adult obesity from 1985 to 2003. The authors provide little commentary on the data they present except to say that:

> The prevalences of overweight and all levels of obesity in Canada have increased between 1985 and 2003 . . . The increases in prevalence of over-weight and all levels of obesity in Canada between 1985 and 2003 are cause for concern given the markedly increased risk of premature death and of met-abolic and musculoskeletal complications arising from morbid obesity. The rapid increase in the prevalences of class II and III obesity will undoubtedly have a significant impact on our health care system.
>
> (Katzmarzyk and Mason 2006: 157)

However, the accompanying data for Canadians (see Figure 3.5) clearly show that adult overweight prevalence was essentially unchanged from 1994 (34.5%) to 2003 (33.9%). From 1994 to 2003 the increase in all categories of obesity (that is, all those with a BMI above 30) was from 13.6% to 15.7% and increased by only 0.8% from 1998 (14.9%) to 2003 (15.7%). A similar levelling-out emerges for all classes of obesity from about 1996 or 1998 onwards. (Class 1 obesity is a BMI between 30.0 and 34.9, Class II between 35.0 and 39.9, and Class III 40 and above.) None of this appears to have been considered worthy of mention by the

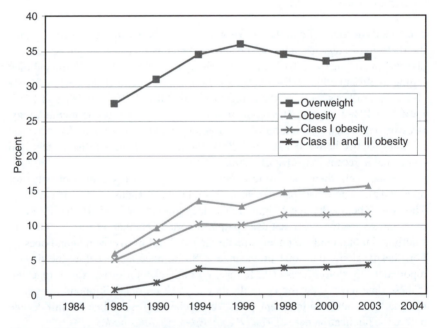

Figure 3.5 Prevalence of overweight and obesity (classes I–III) in Canada, 1985–2003

Source: Adapted from Katzmarzyk and Mason (2006)

authors, presumably because it complicates the story of inexorable increase that they apparently wanted to tell.

More recently, some media reports suggest that Canadian obesity rates have been falling, at least in particular parts of the country. For example, in 2008 The Canadian Press announced 'B.C. [the province of British Columbia] has lowest obesity levels in 10 years' (CTV News 2008). The report is based on the results of the ongoing Canadian Community Health Survey, a data set that is as close to a definitive national survey as currently exists. My source for these data was the Statistics Canada (www.statcan.gc.ca) website, a service that generates longitudinal comparisons using data from a variety of sources.

According to Statistics Canada, the prevalence of Canadian adults with a BMI above 30.0 (obese) was 12.7% in 1994–1995 and 16.0% in 2007, a modest 3.3% increase. Of course, this masks a great deal of diversity across geographic, socio-economic and ethnic groupings. Following on from the press reports about British Columbia, adults in this province recorded an obesity prevalence of 10.2% in 1994–1995, rising to 11.9% in 2000–2001 and down to 11.5% in 2007. This represents an increase of just 1.3% in obesity prevalence over the thirteen-year span of the data set. Of the other provinces, all record higher absolute rates of obesity than British Columbia, although some appear to be increasing while others are essentially stable. For example, adult obesity in Newfoundland and Labrador rose from 20.2% in 2000–2001 to 22% in 2007, but was little changed in Nova Scotia (20.4% to 20.1%) and Manitoba (17.2% to 17.8%) during the same period.

As with any large data set, smaller sub-sets could be excised to show a wide variety of trends in different social sub-groups. However, to describe Canada as a whole as in the grip of an unchecked, ongoing and across-the-board obesity crisis is simply to misrepresent the data that exist.

England and Scotland

Some readers will object to the way I approached obesity data in the previous section. In particular, there will be those who point out that I have relied heavily on aggregated data rather than spending more time looking at cultural or socio-economic sub-groups. However, it is important to be clear that I am attempting to compare readily available, mainstream medical and health data with the obesity rhetoric with which most of us are familiar. It should not be necessary to drill very far down into obesity statistics if, as is alleged, we have a major health emergency on our hands. We need to remember that the mainstream obesity science view is that obesity levels are out of control, represent a global health crisis and affect all levels of Western societies: old and young, black and white, male and female, rich and poor. In other words, if the claims of obesity rhetoric are not borne out in aggregated overweight and obesity statistics then the rhetoric is probably suspect.

The most widely cited trend statistics for body weight in Britain come from the Health Survey for England (HSE). Longitudinal overweight and obesity data from the HSE (and existing previous studies) for adults aged between sixteen and sixty-four years are presented in Table 3.1.

Table 3.1 Body Mass Index prevalence for English adults aged sixteen to sixty-four years

BMI	1986/7 %	1991/92 %	1993 %	1994 %	1995 %	1996 %	1997 %	1998 %	1999 %	2000 %	2001 %	2002 %	2003 %	2004 %
Men														
<20	6	6	5	5	4	4	4	4	5	5	4	5	4	5
20–25	49	41	38	37	36	35	34	34	33	30	28	30	29	29
25–30	38	40	44	44	44	45	45	46	44	45	47	43	44	44
>30	7	13	13	14	15	16	17	17	19	21	21	22	23	23
Women														
<20	11	9	7	7	7	7	7	7	7	6	6	6	6	6
20–25	53	50	44	44	43	41	40	40	39	39	38	37	37	36
25–30	24	26	32	31	33	34	33	32	33	34	33	34	33	35
>30	12	15	16	17	18	18	20	21	21	21	24	23	23	24

Source: Adapted from British Heart Foundation (2009)

These data are striking in the context of claims that British overweight and obesity are increasing rapidly. For example, overweight (BMI between 25 and 30) amongst English men hardly changed at all between 1986–1987 and 2004. In fact, 44% of English men were overweight in 1993; this is exactly the percentage reported in 2004. An almost identical situation existed with women: 32% of women were overweight in 1993 and this was very little changed at 35% in 2004.

In these data the decline in the percentage of 'normal' weight people (BMI 20 and 25) is roughly matched by increases in the number classified as obese (BMI over 30). But here, like prevalence statistics in the United States, it seems that obesity stalled amongst women around the turn of the century. There appears to have been no change at all between 2001 and 2004 and, actually, only a small rise from 21% to 24% between 1998 and 2004. Similarly for men, obesity rose by only 2% (from 21% to 23%) between 2000 and 2004.

More recent HSE data (Health Survey for England 2008a) show these trends for adult overweight and obesity continuing up to the 2008 survey (see Figure 3.6).

For both overweight and obesity it is difficult to see significant changes from 2001 onwards. This point is confirmed, albeit hesitantly, by the survey report authors:

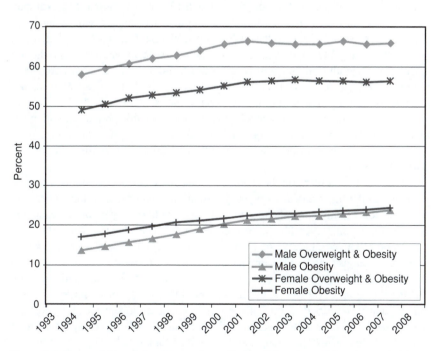

Figure 3.6 Overweight and obesity prevalence for English males and females aged sixteen to sixty-four years, 1993–2008

Source: Adapted from Health Survey for England (2008a)

The proportion who were categorised as obese (BMI 30kg/m2 or over) increased from 13% of men in 1993 to 24% in 2008 and from 16% of women in 1993 to 25% in 2008. However, the rate of increase in obesity prevalence has been slower in the second half of the period than the first half, and there are indications that the trend may be flattening out, at least temporarily. However, it is too soon to tell whether there continues to be a very gradual upward trend, with obesity in women in 2008 at its highest level since 1993 (though not significantly different from 2007). Among men, the proportion who were overweight or obese (BMI 25kg/m^2 or more) increased from 58% in 1993 to 68% in 2001, since when it has fluctuated between 65% and 67% each year, being 66% in 2008. Similarly, the proportion of women who were overweight or obese increased from 49% in 1993 to 57% in 2001, fluctuating at around this level since then; it was 57% in 2008. This pattern therefore broadly matches the pattern for obesity.

(Health Survey for England 2008a: 188–189)

In 2006, England's National Centre for Social Research produced *Forecasting Obesity to 2010*, a report prepared for the Department of Health. It drew on 2003 HSE data and projected these forward to calculate overweight and obesity prevalence for adults and children in the year 2010. These predictions make interesting reading in light of the 2008 report from which I have just quoted. For example, *Forecasting Obesity to 2010* predicted that English adult male obesity would rise from 22% in 2003 to 33% in 2010 (Zaninotto, Wardle, Stamatakis, Mindell and Head 2006: Table 14). In other words, based on the data above, for this prediction to come true, adult male obesity would need to jump by nearly ten percentage points in three years, from 24% in 2007 to 33% in 2010. For women, *Forecasting Obesity to 2010* estimated that obesity would rise from 23% in 2003 to 28% in 2010. As with adult males, it seems highly unlikely that this prediction will eventuate. The data above show that obesity amongst English women appears to have varied in a narrow 1% range between 2001 and 2007, not getting above 24% during this period.

Is it unfair to comment on these apparent inaccuracies? Is this simply a case of being wise after the event, drawing on information to which the earlier forecasters had no access? In my view, the idea that obesity would simply go on increasing at historically unusual rates for the foreseeable future was always extremely dubious – a point Jan Wright and I made over five years ago in *The Obesity Epidemic*. These predictions struck me as unwise then as they do now.

Putting the actual numbers to one side, I am also taken by the gentle lines on the previous graph. And yet, in the first years of the twenty-first century England was regularly described as one of the fattest countries in the Western world, a place where obesity was 'sky rocketing', 'exploding' and, as we saw in Chapter 2, predicted to reach 40% amongst adults by 2025 and 60% by 2050. Without too many years having passed since they were made, I think it is reasonable to ask whether these predictions served any positive purpose. Similarly, I do not think it is mean-spirited hindsight to wonder how so many obesity experts appear to have made the same mistake.

For English children we turn also to the 2008 results from the HSE (Health Survey for England 2008b). The HSE is one of the very few sources of longitudinal overweight and obesity data for English children. Its 2008 version includes the data presented in Figure 3.7 and is explained in the report as follows:

> Between 1995 and 2008, the prevalence of obesity among boys aged 2–15 increased from 11% to 17%, and the equivalent increase for girls was from 12% to 15%. However, the pattern has not been one of uniform increase over the period. The prevalence of obesity increased steadily in most years up to around 2004 and 2005, and since then the pattern has been slightly different for boys and girls. Among boys, the proportion who were obese has remained between 17% and 19% since 2002. Among girls, there was a significant decrease in obesity between 2005 and 2006, and levels have been similar from 2006 to 2008. These results suggest that the trend in obesity now appears to be flattening out, and future HSE data will be important in confirming whether this is a continuing pattern, or whether the longer term trend is still gradually increasing.
>
> (Health Survey England 2008b: 19)

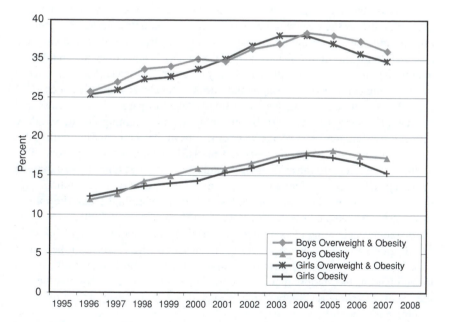

Figure 3.7 Overweight and obesity prevalence for English children aged two to fifteen years by sex, 1995–2008

Source: Adapted from Health Survey for England (2008b)

It is reasonable, I think, to at least question whether a 3% increase (12% to 15%) in the prevalence of girls obesity between 1995 and 2007 represents either an epidemic or a crisis in childhood obesity. In fact, from 1998 to 2008 the rise was from 14% to 15%. While the increase in boys is double this at 6%, it is still only about a 50% increase in twelve years as opposed to the 'doublings' and 'triplings' about which we hear and read. In fact, drawing on the raw numbers that are the basis for this chart, boys' obesity was 17% in 1999, the same percentage reported in 2008 with only small fluctuations between these two points. Whether readers see this as fair comment or not, the pattern here does seem to match the US data we saw in the previous section, with childhood obesity levels flattening out in the period between 2000 and 2004. According to the graph, overweight *and* obesity for girls were both essentially the same in 2007 as they were in 2001, a situation that was only very slightly different for boys.

Turning once again to *Forecasting Obesity to 2010*, obesity for boys was expected to go from 17% in 2003 to 19% in 2010 (Zaninotto, Wardle, Stamatakis, Mindell and Head 2006: Table 15). Here the report appears to have been reasonably accurate, although on current trends even this quite conservative prediction still seems likely to be an overestimate. The corresponding forecast for girls was that obesity would rise from 16% in 2003 to 22% in 2010. Figure 3.7 shows girls' obesity trending slightly downwards and at about 15% in 2007.

Some of the reports discussed so far in this chapter have received media attention because their findings obviously contradict the rhetoric of an epidemic. But this is not always the case with noteworthy obesity statistics. Sometimes significant findings are noticed neither by the media nor, apparently, even the researchers responsible for the findings. For example, Stamatakis and colleagues published longitudinal data on overweight and obesity amongst English children in order to 'examine the childhood overweight and obesity prevalence trends between 1974 and 2003 and to assess whether these trends relate to parental social class and household income' (2005: 999). In this study, data concerning 28,601 children between five and ten years of age were drawn from the National Study of Health and Growth (1974, 1984 and 1994) and the HSE (conducted yearly from 1996 to 2003). According to the authors of the study '. . . these results showed that the upward trends in overweight and obesity in children noted by other authors over the 1990s are continuing into the 2000s and, more alarmingly, that the rate of increase has accelerated over the last decade' (Stamatakis et al. 2005: 1002). The claim about accelerating rates of increase sits alongside Figures 3.8 and 3.9.

In Figure 3.8 the prevalence of obesity amongst English children is broken down to show rates for boys and girls from high- and low-income families. Contrary to the claim of the authors that childhood obesity rates are accelerating, the figure appears to show relatively stable or even downward obesity trends for high-income boys and girls.

With socio-economic differences in mind, the researchers also considered whether parental income or occupation was a better predictor of disparity in childhood obesity. Based on the same data set, Figure 3.9 shows childhood obesity rates for boys and girls from families in which the main income earner had a manual

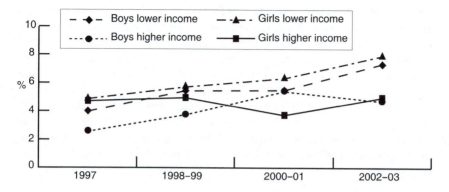

Figure 3.8 Obesity prevalence trends from 1997 to 2002–2003 by income category and sex

Source: Reproduced with permission from Stamatakis et al. (2005)

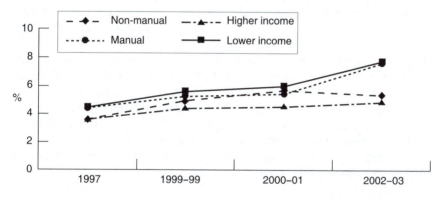

Figure 3.9 Obesity prevalence trends from 1997 to 2002–2003 by income group and social class for boys and girls combined

Source: Reproduced with permission from Stamatakis et al. (2005)

or non-manual job. Like the first, this figure suggests reasonably wide (and, it seems, widening) gaps between children of different social strata, but also steady or declining obesity rates for children from non-manual families.

Stamatakis and colleagues do not report the raw data for these graphs in the published paper, although I have contacted one of the paper's authors and requested the data points. While I do not have permission to reproduce them here, taken together they suggest to me that there was no change at all in obesity levels amongst high-income children (boys and girls aggregated together) between 1998–1999 and 2002–2003. Obesity amongst high-income girls began to decline after 1998–1999 and after 2000–2001 for boys.

Taken together, what is most striking about these findings is that these apparent declines drew no comment whatsoever from the paper's authors. This seems an extraordinary omission. What appears to be a complex and yet intriguing set of results is simply glossed over by the researchers presumably because they could not or did not want to see the good news in their own results. According to these data, since 1997 the difference in the obesity rates of richer and poorer children appears to have grown significantly. To me, these results suggest a number of possible interpretations and future research directions, each of which relate to apparently opposite trends in the obesity rates of richer and poorer English children. Stamatakis and colleagues, though, head off in a different direction, concluding their paper almost as if they are talking about a different data set from the one they have presented:

> Obesity rates among both boys and girls increased at accelerating rates into the early 2000s and these upward trends were more marked among children from lower income families and to a lesser extent among children from manual social classes. Considering the calamitous consequences of obesity, there is an urgent need for action to halt and reverse this rapid upward trend among English children, especially among those from lower socioeconomic strata.
>
> (Stamatakis et al. 2005: 1003)

Apart from anything else, given that the authors call for 'urgent' action, it is curious that Stamatakis and colleagues do not even stop to ask whether anything can be learnt from the apparently stabilising trends for more affluent children.

Elsewhere in Britain, Mitchell, McDougall and Crum (2007) have reported declining rates of obesity in small samples (approximately 350 per cohort) of grade one primary school children in the Scottish city of Aberdeen.

While rates of childhood obesity in Scotland appear to be higher than those of England, the authors of this study concluded that:

> There is a clear downward trend in the prevalence of obesity over the period studied. In 1997, the prevalence of obesity was 14.7%, decreasing to 11.4% in 2001. The figure for 2004 has decreased even further to 10.2%. This trend was present in boys and girls when assessed separately.
>
> (Mitchell, McDougall and Crum 2007: 153)

These data are particularly interesting in the context of widespread comment within Scotland that positions Scottish people as the fattest in Britain and even the fattest in Europe. And while it would it be an obvious mistake to draw too much from Mitchell and colleagues' small study, there are other data that suggest that theirs is not a completely idiosyncratic finding. For example, as far back as the *Scottish Health Survey 2003* we find the following:

> There was an increase, among boys, between 1998 and 2003 in the prevalence of overweight including obesity (from 28.8% to 34.6%), and obesity (from

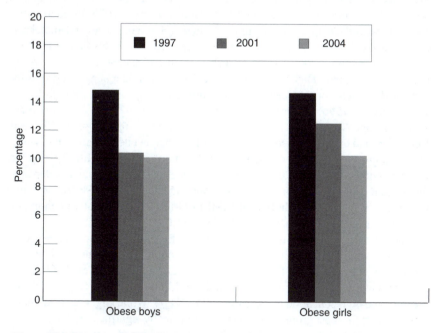

Figure 3.10 Prevalence of obesity for boys and girls

Source: Reproduced with permission from Mitchell et al. (2007)

14.4% to 18.0%). There was no change in girls' overweight or obesity levels between the two years.

(Scottish Government 2005: 110)

More recently, the *Scottish Health Survey 2008* has confirmed this trend:

The increase in the proportion of boys outwith the healthy weight range is accounted for by a corresponding increase in the proportion who were overweight or obese, rather than significant changes in the prevalence of underweight. 27.8% of boys aged 2–15 were overweight in 1998, compared with 32.4% in 2003 and 36.1% in 2008. There were no significant changes among girls aged 2–15 in this period.

(Scottish Government 2009: 201)

The 1998, 2003 and 2008 combined overweight and obesity prevalences for Scottish girls were 28.3%, 28.9% and 26.9% respectively.

Europe

Although most of the studies discussed in this chapter have appeared only in the last couple of years, we do not have to look particularly hard to find earlier evidence that obesity was never quite an all-pervasive global contagion. A Danish study that tracked obesity prevalence in about 30, 000 adults from the 1970s through to the 1990s found little support for the epidemic thesis (Heitmann, Strøger, Mikkelsen, Holst and Sørensen 2004). Overall, the study reported that obesity had either been stable or declining amongst most Danish women and increasing only in some age cohorts of men. This finding followed Norwegian data suggesting obesity increased in men but declined amongst women from the 1960s through to the 1980s (Tverdal 1996). Reporting on the period between 1972 and 1992, Pietinen, Vartiainen and Männistö (1996) found that obesity amongst Finnish men aged forty years and over increased from 1972 to 1987 but levelled off after that, while obesity amongst women decreased until 1982 and then levelled off. This study, like many others since, also found large differences in obesity prevalence depending on educational levels. In Sweden, Lissner and colleagues (1998) found some increase in waist-hip ratio but not in BMI in different representative cohorts of women measured in 1968–1969, 1980–1981 and 1992–1993.

A small but growing number of more recent European studies have reported overweight and obesity prevalence trends that contradict the general picture of a rapidly worsening crisis. For Swiss adults, Wolff and colleagues (2006) have compared obesity prevalence for approximately 13,000 males and females of low, medium and high education levels from 1993 to 2004. While slight upward trends were evident for most groups, there was no statistically significant increase at the 0.5 level for any group except men classified as 'medium education' level.

Aeberli, Ammann, Knabenhans, Molinari and Zimmermann (2009) have reported a comparison of two surveys of Swiss children aged between six and thirteen years. The surveys measured the heights and weights of 2,431 children in 2002 and 2,222 in 2007 to produce two nationally representative samples. The researchers reported a statistically significant decline in mean BMI across the two surveys from 17.7 to 17.4 for all children. In addition:

> The prevalence of underweight has not changed significantly over the 5 years, but the prevalences of overweight and obesity have decreased. For boys, the decrease in overweight [12.5% to 11.5%] was not significant ($P = 0.37$), but for girls [13.2% to 10.0%] it was ($P < 0.01$). For obesity, the decrease was significant in both boys [7.4% to 5.3%] ($P = 0.049$) and girls [5.7% to 3.3%] ($P < 0.01$).
>
> (Aeberli et al. 2009: 3)

If we assume that the findings of this study are real, they raise the question of whether the decline began before or after the year 2002. The authors of this study make what appears to me to be the mistake of claiming that Swiss childhood overweight and obesity increased up until the 2002 and then declined thereafter. They write, 'Our findings suggest the increasing prevalence of childhood overweight and obesity in Switzerland until 2002 may be coming under control' (Aeberli, Ammann, Knabenhans, Molinari and Zimmermann 2009: 5). There is no reason to assume that the reversal of previous increases did not begin prior to or, alternatively, following 2002. Both are possibilities. In fact, it seems most unlikely that the researchers managed to time their data collection periods perfectly to coincide with the turning of the tide.

As with most of the studies presented in this chapter, it seems to me more likely that the reversal of previous upward trends began before, not after, the time of the first data collection point. Taking this Swiss study as an example, if childhood overweight and obesity were still going up in 2002, then the subsequent reversal of this trend would need to have been very rapid indeed, fast enough to wipe off all of the post-2002 increases *as well as* to drop below 2002 levels by 2007. We should remember also that this study does not report trend reversals in one group, say obese girls, and not others. All groups – boys and girls and overweight and obese – showed no increase after 2002 and all groups except overweight boys show a decline. In other words, the trend reported here appears to be widespread rather than piecemeal, a situation which is more likely to be explained by a longer and more gradual reversal rather than a shorter and sharper one. Trends in male and female body weight generally lag one another, rarely moving up and down at exactly the same time. So, if the body weight of both Swiss boys and girls were both trending upwards at some point prior to 2002, it would have taken some length of time for them both to start heading in the opposite direction. Of course, it is impossible to be sure about any of this but, on balance, it seems more plausible that Aeberli and colleagues' data reflect a gradual trend of first flattening and then declining childhood overweight and obesity that was at least underway prior to 2002.

To take another example, Romon and colleagues' (2008) study in *Public Health Nutrition* shows combined overweight and obesity for primary school children declining in two small French towns from at least the year 2000. This study collected measurements from a majority of the children living in these two towns for the years 1992, 2000, 2002, 2003 and 2004, with yearly samples varying in size from about 600 to about 800 children. Using the term 'overweight' to include all overweight and obese five- to twelve-year-olds in their study, they concluded:

> Between 1992 and 2000, there was an increase in BMI and overweight prevalence. From 2000 to 2004, there was a decrease in the prevalence of overweight which was more pronounced in girls. For girls and boys taken together, the overweight prevalence was 13.2% (sixty-eight children), 10.5 % (sixty-two children) and 8.8% (fifty-six children) in 2002, 2003 and 2004, respectively. For the same years, the prevalence was 9.5%, 7.7% and 7.4% for the boys and 17.1 %, 13.6% and 10.4 % for the girls. When the years 1992 and 2004 are compared, there was no significant difference in the prevalence of overweight for either boys or girls.
>
> (Romon et al. 2008: 1737)

Strictly speaking, the researchers are correct to say that their study recorded an increase in overweight and obesity from 1992 to 2000, but this does not rule out the possibility that that the downward trend started before 2000.

Similarly, Peneau, Salanave, Rolland-Cachera, Hercberg and Castetbon (2009) have presented overweight obesity prevalence data for French children aged between seven and nine years. Using samples of 1,582 children in 2000 and 1,014 in 2007, the researchers found that, combing all children, overweight fell from 18.1% to 15.8% and obesity fell from 3.6% to 2.8%. The corresponding falls for overweight and obesity amongst boys were 17.9% to 14.1% and 3.9% to 2.8% respectively, while prevalences for girls declined from 18.3% to 17.7% and 3.6% to 2.8% respectively. None of these falls reached statistical significance.

Some of the researchers involved in this study have also published 'Prevalence of overweight in 6- to 15-year-old children in central/western France from 1996 to 2006: trends toward stabilization' in the *International Journal of Obesity* (Péneau et al. 2009). This study used data on approximately 26,000 six- to fifteen-year-old children measured between 1996 and 2006. Once again, the term 'overweight' includes children classified as obese:

> An increase in the prevalence of overweight was observed from 1996 to 1998 in boys (10.7–14.1%) and from 1996 to 1999 in girls (12.4–16.3%). Following these dates, the prevalence was generally stable in both groups until the end of the study. On the basis of the linear regression analyses, no significant increase in the prevalence of overweight was observed in either gender over the 1996–2006 period. During the 1996–2001 period, there was an increase in the prevalence of overweight that was statistically significant in boys only. During the 2001–2006 period, the prevalence of overweight was stable in both genders.
>
> (Péneau et al. 2009: 403)

The year 2001 is significant in this study because the researchers were interested in whether the stabilisation of childhood overweight and obesity could be attributed to government initiatives begun in that year. However, they concluded that the stabilisation appears to have happened sometime during 1998–1999.

These findings are similar to those of Lioret and colleagues (2009), who drew on two nationally representative samples of French children (approximately 1,000 per sample) aged between three and fourteen years. Between 1998–1999 and 2006–2007, the study found no statistical change in combined overweight and obesity prevalence. Overweight and obesity were also stable across this period for all age and parental occupational status groupings.

Taken together, these studies suggest there has been very little change in overweight and obesity prevalence amongst French children for ten years or more.

With respect to French adults, Czernichow and colleagues (2009) have analysed data collected in Social Security Health Examination Centres in the central-western region of the country. Drawing on measurements of about 340,000 French men and women, they found increasing obesity prevalence in some socio-economic groups between 1995 and 2005. However, men and women classified as 'management professionals' and men classified as 'office/service personnel' showed no increase during this ten-year period. In addition, both male and female office/service personnel and 'manual worker' women were stable between 2001 and 2005. Overall, the study reported that 6.9% of men and 6.4% of women were obese in 1995 and 8.9% and 8.6% respectively in 2005. These prevalence rates are less than one-third of those reported in the US.

Rana, Herman and Stefaan (2009) have analysed the results of the three large surveys, in 1997, 2001 and 2004, of Belgian women and men over eighteen years of age. This study was primarily interested in whether increasing levels of obesity were affecting Belgians differently according to socio-economic status. Using educational level as a proxy for socio-economic status, the researchers found, in keeping with earlier research, that highly educated Belgian women were much less likely than less educated women to be obese, although the socio-economic gap did not appear to be increasing over time. The gap was smaller between high- and low-educated men, but it was widening and catching up to women. Interesting also, female obesity increased between 1997 and 2004 (8.98% to 10.93%), but it was unchanged for men (9.60% to 9.99%). In fact, while obesity prevalence amongst men with lower education levels increased, it fell amongst more educated men.

The results of a Dutch study (de Wilde, van Dommelen, Middelkoop and Verkerk 2009) covering the period from 1999 to 2007 and using data from just over 50,000 three- to sixteen-year-old children lend more support to the widely reported conclusion that trends in childhood obesity, like many other social variables, diverge significantly according to ethnicity in Western countries. Large differences in overweight and obesity prevalence percentages were found, from least to most overweight and obese, for children from Dutch, Surinamese, Moroccan and Turkish backgrounds. There was a non-significant change in obesity for Dutch boys (2.2% to 2.3%) and a significant decline for girls (3.7% to 3.3%). The authors of the study also concluded:

> From 1999 through 2007 there was a decrease in the prevalence of overweight [excluding obesity] in Dutch girls from 12.6% to 10.9% and an increase in Turkish boys from 14.6% to 21.4%. Obesity prevalence rose significantly in Turkish boys from 7.9% to 13.1% and in Turkish girls from 8.0% to 10.7%. Dutch boys, and Moroccan and Surinamese South Asian boys and girls showed no significant trends.
>
> (de Wilde et al. 2009: 795)

In the case of Sweden, a small collection of published studies paints a similar picture. In their article 'Childhood overweight and obesity prevalences leveling off in Stockholm but socioeconomic differences persist' for the *International Journal of Obesity*, Sundblom, Petzold, Rasmussen, Callmer and Lissner (2008) compared two samples of ten-year-old children from Stockholm county. The first was in 1999 (2,416 children) and the second was in 2003 (2,183 children). Between 1999 and 2003, boys' overweight fell from 21.6% to 20.5% while obesity rose from 3.2% to 3.8%. Girls' overweight decreased from 22.1% to 19.2 % and obesity decreased from 4.4% to 2.8%. These results translated into a marginally statistically significant fall in obesity for ten-year-old girls, but there was no significant change in the other categories.

These findings are similar to another group of Swedish researchers, also reporting data for ten-year-old children, but this time in the city of Gothenburg (Sjöberg, Lissner, Albertsson-Wikland and Mårild 2008). The study measured 4,683 children in 2000–2001 and 4,193 in 2004–2005, finding that:

> Between 2000/2001 and 2004/2005, the prevalence of overweight plus obesity in girls decreased from 19.6% to 15.9% (p < 0.01). Prevalence of obesity was 3.0% and 2.5% (nonsignificant), respectively. In boys, all differences between the corresponding cohorts were nonsignificant: 17.1% versus 17.6% were overweight (including obese) and 2.9% versus 2.8% were obese.
>
> (Sjöberg et al. 2008: 118)

New Zealand

In 2008 the New Zealand Ministry of Health released *A Portrait of Health: Key Results of the 2006/07 New Zealand Health Survey* (Ministry of Health 2008). The 2006–2007 New Zealand Health Survey sampled 12,488 adults and 4,921 children and, for the purposes of historical comparison, was analysed against the 1997 National Nutrition Survey and the 2002 National Children's Nutrition Survey.

Despite receiving a huge amount of publicity, obesity prevalence amongst adults in New Zealand is commensurate with countries such as England while lagging behind the United States (see Figure 3.11). The authors of *A Portrait of Health* comment:

> There has been an increase in the prevalence of obesity for [all] men and [all] women from 1997 to 2006/07, adjusted for age. However, the rate of increase appears to be slowing, with no statistically significant increase between 2002/03 and 2006/07 for both men and women.
>
> (Ministry of Health 2008: 117)

While much higher than non-Māori New Zealanders, *A Portrait of Health* reports an even earlier plateau for Māori adults: 'For Māori adults there was no significant change from 1997 to 2006/07 in the prevalence of obesity for both men and women, adjusted for age' (Ministry of Health 2008: 118). The accompanying graph is difficult to square with predictions that Māori are heading towards an obesity-driven extinction.

A Portrait of Health presents two sets of results for childhood obesity, one for the general population and one for Māori, both of which show no change for the 2002 to 2006–2007 interval. In fact, for Māori girls, Māori boys and all girls, statistically non-significant declines were recorded, while the statistic for all boys was steady at 10%.

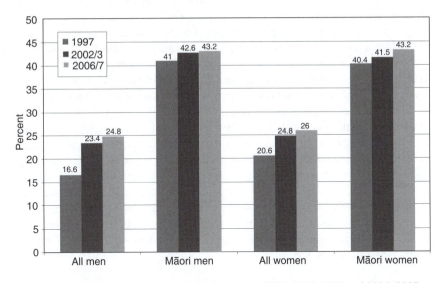

Figure 3.11 Obesity prevalence for adults, by gender, 1997, 2002–2003 and 2006–2007

Source: Adapted from Ministry of Health (2008)

We do not have the luxury of comparing a range of data sets concerning longitudinal overweight and obesity trends in New Zealand – a problem it shares with many other Western countries. No single set of research findings is beyond

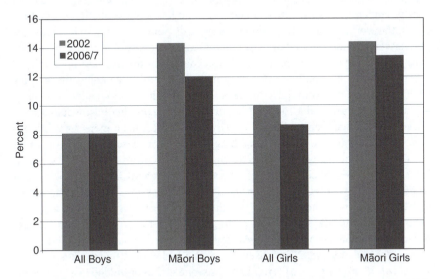

Figure 3.12 Obesity prevalence for children aged five to fourteen years, by gender, 2002 and 2006–2007

Source: Adapted from Ministry of Health (2008)

question or dispute and I certainly do not want to suggest that these data – or any other study for any other country – is the end of the matter. And yet it is surely reasonable to at least take seriously the data that do exist, in this case deriving from research supported by the New Zealand government and conducted by reputable researchers using standard procedures. So, when we read in New Zealand's widely read *Listener* magazine in early 2010 that 'Over the past four decades, the incidence of heart disease and strokes has significantly declined, but as a nation we keep getting fatter' (Johns 2010: 22) and 'We may be moving more but we're still getting fatter' (Clifton 2010: 26), is it sufficient to simply write this off as uninformed journalism? In both of these articles a series of obesity experts are quoted at considerable length about the apparently desperate situation facing New Zealand. More broadly though, while I have heard a number of well-known obesity researchers concede in informal conversation that perhaps too much has been made of obesity, it still appears to be extremely rare for experts to challenge the exaggerations and errors that appear regularly in the media. To put the point bluntly, journalists have not simply made this stuff up; the buck stops with the obesity research community.

Australia

In mid-2009, the Australian Bureau of Statistics released results of the 2007–2008 National Health Survey. The survey found that in the years between 1995 and 2008 combined overweight and obesity for Australian adult males rose from 64% to 68%. For women, the rise was marginally larger: from 49% to 55%. So, according to this national survey, during the period of time in which the idea of an obesity epidemic was first created and then – no less in Australia than anywhere else in the world – regularly described as spiralling out of control, the prevalence of overweight and obese adult males increased, in proportional terms, by a little over 6%. Perhaps even more remarkably, it found that the increase in childhood obesity, the much-remarked upon 'ticking time-bomb' threatening the world's health systems, was from 5.2% to 7.8%. It is difficult not to wonder how many average Australians, fed a constant diet of cataclysmic predictions, would be surprised to learn that their childhood obesity crisis concerned a mere 7.8% of children. Surprise might to turn to something stronger – a sense of betrayal perhaps – when they learn that while obesity amongst boys rose from 4.5% to 9.7%, prevalence for girls remained unchanged at 5.8%. Almost as if he were looking at a completely different set of statistics, the implacably pessimistic Paul Zimmet (see also Chapter 2) was quoted saying that the survey confirmed his belief that 'Our nation's public health planner's need to gear up for the largest chronic disease burden this nation has ever faced' (Australian Science Media Centre 2009).

A recent study by Olds, Tomkinson, Ferrar and Maher (2010) in the *International Journal of Obesity* combined the results of forty-one studies of childhood weight status in Australia published between 1985 and 2008. In essence, this involved converting all the data from these studies into a common measure of childhood overweight and obesity that could then be tracked over time. The authors reported that:

The main findings of this study are that a) the prevalence of overweight and obesity in Australian children has flattened over the last decade or so, b) this trend is fairly consistent across different age groups, and c) within weight status categories, average BMI appears to have plateaued. These findings directly contradict assertions in the published literature and the popular press that the prevalence of pediatric overweight and obesity in Australia is increasing exponentially.

(Olds et al. 2010: 62)

The graphic depiction of this analysis (Figure 3.13) suggests that the flattening of Australian childhood overweight and obesity percentages may have happened prior to the year 2000.

In numerical terms, this analysis estimates that the prevalence of combined overweight and obesity amongst boys was 10.2% in 1985 and 21.6% in 1996, but then rose only to 23.7% in 2008. In girls, the corresponding estimates are 11.6% in 1985, 24.3% in 1996 and 24.8% in 2008. For boys' obesity alone, the study

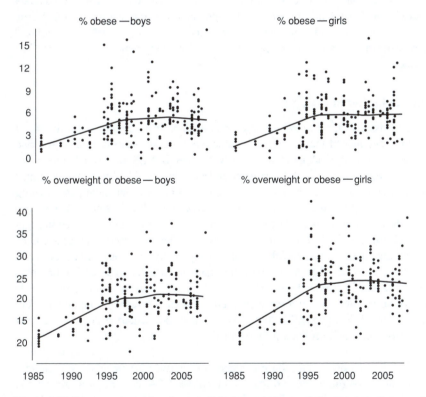

Figure 3.13 Lowess curves showing trends in the prevalence of obesity alone (top panels) and overweight and obesity (bottom panels) for boys (left-hand panels) and girls (right-hand panels)

Source: Reproduced with permission from Olds et al. (2010)

estimated that the prevalence in 1985 was 1.0%, 5.4% in 1996, and still only 5.3% over a decade later in 2008. For girls, the 1985 obesity estimate was 0.8%, rising rapidly to 5.7% in 1996 but then only marginally higher at 5.9% in 2008. In short, the study found that the rate of increase in Australian children's BMI between 1996 and 2008 was less than one-sixth of the rate of increase between 1985 and 1996.

It is true that analyses of this kind involve a good deal of data massaging in order to combine the results of studies that might have used different measurements or reported their data in different ways. Still, this is the only meta-analysis of its kind that I am aware of. And although it is a very different kind of study to the mainly descriptive research that I have considered in this chapter, its findings do bear a striking resemblance to the picture emerging from many other countries. In other words, there is evidence that overweight and obesity prevalence amongst Western children had flattened and, in some cases, begun to decline even before the world-wide alarm about spiralling childhood obesity had been raised. Two of the authors of this study have also completed a review of international childhood obesity data that includes some of the European and US data discussed above as well as data from China, Greenland and Italy (Olds, personal communication 2009). While not yet published, these data also suggest that previous increases in childhood obesity prevalence slowed, stopped or reversed in many countries during the last decade.

The beginning of the end

In a 2005 issue of the *Journal of the American Dietetic Association* Blackburn and Waltman announced that the obesity epidemic, at least in the United States, had stopped in the year 2002. Even at this early stage, NHANES data were beginning to show a leveling out of obesity prevalence and Blackburn and Waltman were amongst the first to notice. However, this was not, and still is not, a widely held view. Writing in the *Journal of the Royal Society for the Promotion of Health*, Walker (2003: 150) posed the question 'The obesity epidemic: is it out of control?' and answered strongly in the affirmative. In the *International Journal of Obesity* Lobstein, James and Cole warned that 'Excess bodyweight in children is widely prevalent in economically developed countries and appears to be increasing in virtually all countries for which data are available' (2003: 1136). More recently, Anderssen and colleagues' assessment of in the international obesity literature was that 'There is no sign that the obesity epidemic is leveling off' (2008: 316). And in a commentary article for *Archives of Disease in Childhood* Thompson claimed:

> There is no doubt that the prevalence of overweight and obesity is rapidly rising throughout the world. Although the USA continues to report the highest national obesity rates, the prevalence of obesity in both developed and developing countries is increasing dramatically and is approaching or matches US rates in some countries.
>
> (2008: 722)

While visiting Australia in 2009, leading obesity researcher Eric Ravussin was quoted in the media saying that, as far as the war on obesity was concerned, there was no good news; nothing was working and no significant progress was being made. For Delpeuch, Maire, Monnier and Holdsworth, 'the obesity epidemic has spread to the whole planet, and nothing seems about to stem its relentless progress' (2009: 6).

As these examples show, the rhetoric of a devastating, uncontrolled and continuously escalating epidemic of obesity survived in academic papers and the mass media well into the first decade of the new century. At the time of writing (early 2010) there were few signs that this situation was changing.

One recent example of a potential shift appeared in late 2009 with the release of *Obesity: Recent trends in children aged 2–11y and 12–19y: Analysis from the Health Survey for England 1993–2007* (McPherson, Brown, Marsh and Byatt 2009). Compiled by The United Kingdom's National Heart Forum, the report compared two sets of predictions for childhood obesity in England. The first set comes from the 2007 Foresight report (see Chapter 2) and is based on HSE data for the years 1993 to 2004. The second set uses data covering the period 2000 to 2007. The report concluded that using more recent data greatly reduced the projected levels of childhood overweight and obesity for the year 2020. In Table 3.2, we see a comparison of the two sets of predictions for males and females aged between two and eleven years and between twelve and nineteen years respectively.

As the table shows, the new predictions have overweight and obesity going down for boy and girls and for all age groupings. In some cases the more recent calculations produce very large discrepancies: the percentage of normal weight 12–19 females rises from 35% to 62%, overweight 2–11 females falls from 34% to 17%, obese 12–19 males falls from 19% to 6% and obese 12–19 females falls precipitously from 30% to 9%. It is worth remembering that in June 2004 David Hinchliffe, Head of Britain's Parliamentary Health Commission, warned that if

Table 3.2 Comparison of childhood overweight and obesity prevalence predictions for 2020

Predictions to 2020	Foresight 1993–2004	2000–2007
% Normal weight males 2–11	57	70
% Normal weight females 2–11	52	72
% Overweight males 2–11	22	17
% Overweight females 2–11	34	17
% Obese males 2–11	20	13
% Obese females 2–11	14	10
% Normal weight males 12–19	56	76
% Normal weight females 12–19	35	62
% Overweight males 12–19	25	18
% Overweight females 12–19	35	29
% Obese males 12–19	19	6
% Obese females 12–19	30	9

Source: Adapted from McPherson et al. (2009)

trends continued, 50% of England's children would be obese by 2020 (Delpeuch, Maire, Monnier and Holdsworth 2009: 12). Based on the more recent predictions cited here, rather than 50%, there would appear to be at least a fighting chance that the eventual figure will not even reach double figures.

The obvious point to make is that this is one of the first set of predictions that does not assume that obesity levels will go on rising indefinitely and at rates seen briefly during the 1990s. Furthermore, if the phenomenon of flattening and, in some cases, falling rates of overweight and obesity are a real finding, there is an inescapable conclusion: almost all past predictions about future rates of overweight and obesity, future costs of treating obesity-related disease and the future impact of overweight and obesity on Western life expectancy must now be discounted.

I have already made the point that when obesity experts have claimed that obesity rates were still going up they have invariably been referring to data that were a number of years old. They simply had no way of telling whether obesity was still going up and they were wrong to claim that it was. Although I expect to be accused of splitting hairs, I do not think this is a trivial point since it relates to the precision with which scientists communicate their findings to each other and to the public. Moreover, if Chapter 2 proved nothing else, it is that once exaggerations and half-truths about obesity get running, they are hard to stop.

But as interesting as they are, the imprecisions and exaggerations of obesity science are not the take-home story here. Rather, it is that just as the idea of an obesity epidemic was first being breathlessly thrust upon the world – roughly a couple of years either side of the turn of the century – the phenomenon itself was already in decline.

4   The view from outside

Although the evidence base is very small, some obesity experts argue that Western body weights have been increasing for fifty years; others even suggest that the trend goes back a 100 or 200 years. They may well be right about this, although a large part of this can surely be attributed to the mostly desirable impact of improving living standards. However, my sense is that some obesity experts see this gradual increase in body weights as a creeping, insidious descent into sloth, gluttony and general ill health.

Perhaps the most instructive and bizarre example of this that I have seen is a study by Egger, Vogels and Westerterp (2001), published in the *Medical Journal of Australia*. Apparently with a view to making a point about declining physical activity levels, the researchers selected a group of male actors working at Old Sydney Town, a theme park that attempted to recreate life in a penal colony during the first years of European settlement in Australia. The actors, playing the roles of soldiers, convicts and settlers, went about their colonial business for eight hours a day, were instructed to avoid all modern labour-saving technology and some lived in the theme park's convict huts for four days and nights. The amount of physical activity performed by the theme park workers over the duration of the study was then compared to a group of 'sedentary' urban workers, including doctors, taxi drivers and one 'entertainer'.

It will perhaps surprise few readers that the theme park workers expended significantly more calories than the urban group, although the difference was perhaps not as large one might imagine. The theme park workers were 1.6 times more active than the urban workers. However, the researchers decided that two particularly committed theme park workers 'who kept rigidly to the experimental requirements' (Egger, Vogels and Westerterp 2001: 636) provided a more realistic comparison. These two individuals were 2.3 times more active than the modern group – a difference, according to the researchers, of walking about sixteen kilometres per day.

What significance should we draw from these results? I actually visited Old Sydney Town as a child and recall little about the lifestyle of its 'residents' that struck me as healthy or worthy of emulation. But for Egger, Vogels and Westerterp:

These findings support the suggestion that, if the evolutionary perspective (which has dominated almost all of human existence) is indicative of requirements for optimal health, an increase in activity levels up to three times those recommended in modern guidelines may be necessary.

(2001: 636)

In other words, the researchers appear to have seriously entertained the idea that the harsh conditions that existed in early colonial Australia tell us something meaningful about how we should live our modern lives. They conclude by claiming that their findings '. . . add support to other attempts to calculate human activity levels over time and provide an indication of the activity requirements needed to correct these secular changes' (Egger, Vogels and Westerterp 2001: 636). While my contention would be that their data tell us nothing whatsoever about how much physical activity we should do in order to be healthy, Egger, Vogels and Westerterp are clearly of the view that, on some level, the life re-created by their actors offers, as they put it, a 'correction' to the way we live today. This is pure speculation. Just because an early Australian convict may have done a certain amount of physical activity – lets call this amount x – there is absolutely no way of judging what the significance of x is. The extent of Egger, Vogels and Westerterp's argument seems to be that because a convict did more daily exercise than an office worker, we should live more like a convict than an office worker.

While many other examples of obesity researchers waxing nostalgic about the past exist, the central point is that there is an odd paradox at work here. While there could surely be no argument about the superior health of most modern Westerners compared to 100 or 200 years ago, obesity researchers and experts constantly focus on the past when things, they say, were better. As we saw in Chapter 2, in its most extreme form this nostalgia rears its head in statements, like those of Mike Adams, that today's Americans are the most diseased group of people in the history of human civilisation. Although usually less hyperbolic, the obesity research literature is almost uniformly convinced that people lived healthier lives in the past, whether in the caves and on the savannahs of our distant ancestors or in the supposedly crime- and traffic-free suburbs of our parents' and grandparents' generations.

A comparison of present and historical standards of health in Western countries is well beyond the scope of this book. I also do not propose to offer yet another commentary on the health implications of over overweight and obesity. Suffice to say that the matter continues to be vigorously debated and that there are grounds for doubting the idea that fatness, in and of itself, is the killer it is often claimed to be (a growing literature to this effect exists but interested readers could consult Farrell, Braun, Barlow, Cheng and Blair 2002; Orpana et al. 2010; Simpson et al. 2007). My more modest goal in this brief chapter is to share what, for me, has been one of the enduring curiosities of studying obesity.

As we saw in Chapter 2, many obesity researchers and experts think that obesity will lead to a very serious decline in the health of Western populations, a possible decline in life expectancy and will have a serious, if not catastrophic, impact on the viability of health systems and infrastructure around the world. It is for this reason, for example, that obesity researchers have spent so much time trying to calculate the economic costs of rising obesity. In short, this is what we might call the view from inside the obesity epidemic tent. The insiders are a roughly discernable core of researchers, clinicians, public health advocates and other health workers whose work focuses on obesity – people who have taken up the idea of an obesity epidemic (at least as I described it in Chapter 2) as their 'cause' or at least one of their causes. They are the obesity epidemic's 'true believers', if you will.

With this admittedly shadowy group in mind, I want to now consider the view from outside the obesity tent. How serious does the obesity epidemic look to people who need to think about health issues other than obesity or, in fact, the general health of entire populations? Do they see obesity as a looming health tsunami, a threat equivalent to global warming or a destructive force powerful enough to undo the public health gains of the past?

In making a comparison between the obesity epidemic tent's insiders and outsiders, I will say little about whose opinion we should put most faith in. No doubt there are arguments for siding with those on the hard-core and committed inside and arguments for going with less feverish outsiders, although readers will have little trouble guessing where my sympathies are likely to lie. In fact, over the remainder of this chapter I do not expect to win any arguments or radically change readers' minds. Instead, I have kept this chapter deliberately short because I understand how contentious, exhausting and, from time to time, fruitless debates about the heath risks of fatness can be. What I offer here is simply a small morsel of food for thought: given the intensity of insiders' rhetoric, why do those on the outside talk in more measured terms, positioning obesity as just one of the many health issues that Western nations face? In other words, even if readers are inclined to dismiss the views of doubters like me, what are we to make of the generally rosy health picture painted by senior health officials from many countries that are, the obesity insiders say, in the midst of a deepening and catastrophic obesity crisis?

This is one of the enduring curiosities of obesity research that I mentioned above: why is the view inside the obesity epidemic tent so apparently different from the view outside? For now, I leave readers to their private thoughts on the matter. What follows is a brief sample of governmental reports on the health of a small group of Western nations. My sample is limited for two reasons. First, I wish only to exemplify the phenomenon that interests me and to avoid labouring the point. Second, a similar story emerges no matter where one looks around the Western industrialised world.

The United States

In early 2010 I was one of six invited speakers at a lively obesity-focused conference in New Zealand. During a Q&A session at the end of the conference an audience member asked the six speakers to say, in turn, whether they thought obesity was a disease. In a scene that weirdly echoed the famous April 1994 United States Congressional Hearing (in which a group of seven tobacco industry executives said, one-by-one, that no, nicotine was not addictive) all six of us said no, obesity was not a disease. However, one of the group, a professor from a world-leading medical research institution, offered the caveat that, while obesity may not be a disease itself, there certainly was 'more disease around' and that obesity was probably playing a role.

At the time, I baulked at asking the professor what they meant by 'more disease'. It had been a draining couple of days, full of argument and counter-argument and the post-conference drinks beckoned. Still, it would have been interesting to inquire if this comment amounted to a claim that more people were getting sick more often – what I presumed it to mean – or something else.

At the risk of putting words in someone else's mouth, the idea that there is more disease around appears to echo Egger, Vogels and Westerterp (and many other obesity researchers), that people living in Western societies today are sicker and less healthy than they were in the past. This is clearly the kind of broad generalisation that is difficult to prove or disprove. At the same time, there is no shortage of sources to consult that might at least help us to judge whether the claim is plausible.

For example, in 2009 the US Department of Health and Human Services released *Health, United States, 2008* (National Center for Health Statistics 2009), a 590-page report on the state of American health. If there is more disease around it is not a claim that is substantiated or even made in this report. On the contrary, to the extent that death itself is a measure of how much sickness there is, it is not at all clear that things are getting worse:

> In 2005, a total of 2.4 million deaths were reported in the United States. The overall age-adjusted death rate was 45% lower in 2005 than in 1950. The reduction in overall mortality since 1950 was driven mostly by declines in mortality for such leading causes of death as heart disease, stroke, and unintentional injuries. In 2005, the age-adjusted death rate for heart disease, the leading cause of death, was 64% lower than the rate in 1950. The age-adjusted death rate for stroke, the third leading cause of death, declined 74% since 1950.
>
> (National Center for Health Statistics 2009: 50)

Of course, that people are staying alive longer does not mean that fewer people are getting sick. Some improvements in mortality are the result of modern medicine's ability to keep sick people alive. Still, researchers who study disease, their risk factors and mortality rates generally argue that historical improvements are the combined result of medical technology and improved lifestyles (Bennett et al. 2006; Gregg et al. 2005; Gregg and Guralnik 2007; McCarron, Davey Smith and Okasha 2002). At any rate, American life expectancy has risen throughout the period of increasing obesity: 'In 2006, American men could expect to live 3.6 years longer, and women 1.9 years longer, than they did in 1990. Mortality from heart disease, stroke, and cancer has continued to decline in recent years' (National Center for Health Statistics 2009: 3). In fact, life expectancy increased more for black Americans than white Americans even though obesity affects black people more than white people:

> Between 1990 and 2006, life expectancy at birth increased more for the black than for the white population, thereby narrowing the gap in life expectancy between these two racial groups. In 1990, life expectancy at birth for the white population was 7.0 years longer than for the black population. By 2006, the difference had narrowed to 4.9 years.
>
> (National Center for Health Statistics 2009: 9)

The document's executive summary includes one paragraph on obesity, a health issue that, elsewhere, obesity experts regularly describe as being as serious as smoking, dwarfing all other health problems:

> Of concern for all Americans is the high prevalence of people with risk factors such as obesity and insufficient exercise, which are associated with chronic diseases such as heart disease, diabetes, and hypertension. Obesity rates do not appear to be increasing as rapidly as they did in past decades, but remain at unacceptable levels with over one-third of adults age 20 and over considered to be obese in 2005–2006.
>
> (National Center for Health Statistics 2009: 4)

Notice here that there is little to suggest the situation is getting worse. The document's authors think obesity prevalence is 'unacceptable', but the rhetoric of galloping rates of overweight and obesity is absent. It would perhaps be nit-picking to pounce on the claim that obesity is not 'increasing as rapidly' as previous decades when, in fact, research findings suggest that American obesity rates may not have been increasing at all by 2006 (see Chapter 3). Still, what we have here appears to be obesity more as a public health irritant than a disaster.

Some obesity experts concede that life expectancy has improved in recent decades, but they counter by saying that, while we are living longer, we are living fewer sickness-free years and are being kept alive by improvements in medical technology. Although only relatively recent data are available, *Health, United States, 2008* offers little support for this view:

> Between 1997 and 2006, the percentage of non-institutionalized working-age adults 18–64 years of age reporting an activity limitation caused by a chronic health condition remained relatively stable . . . (42) [And later] Between 1997 and 1999, the percentage of non-institutionalized adults 65 years and over with limitation of activity decreased. Between 2000 and 2006, the percentage was relatively stable.
>
> (National Center for Health Statistics 2009: 44)

In addition, the age-adjusted percentage of Americans reporting fair or poor health was 9.2 % in 2006, slightly down from 10.4% in 1991. Even without adjusting for age and the higher proportion of older people in the population, the percentage was 10% in 1991 and only 9.5% in 2006.

Mirroring trends around the world, American rates of heart disease mortality have fallen precipitously in recent decades, while cancer mortality has also dropped:

> Age-adjusted mortality from heart disease, the leading cause of death overall, declined 38% between 1990 and 2006, continuing a long-term downward trend. Age-adjusted mortality from cancer (malignant neoplasms), the second leading cause of death overall, decreased 16% between 1990 and 2006.
>
> (National Center for Health Statistics 2009: 9)

The long-term trend is striking indeed. In 1950, the age-adjusted death rate for heart diseases was 586.8 per 100,000 people in 1950 and 211.1 in 2005. Even without adjusting for age, heart disease deaths fell from 355.5 per 100,000 in 1950 to 220 in 2005.

It is perhaps worth noting that many of the statistics quoted here are age adjusted. This qualification is in recognition of the fact that, despite rising levels of overweight and obesity, Americans are living longer. Since diseases such as heart disease and cancer are primarily diseases of aging, a higher proportion of older people in the population potentially means a higher raw, unadjusted prevalence of these diseases. The process of age adjusting seeks to estimate disease prevalence as if there had been no change in the proportion of any age group. After all, lower rates of heart disease amongst younger people is a good outcome that needs to be reflected in heath statistics, despite the fact that it leads to more people surviving into older age when they are statistically more prone to heart disease. It is partly this fact that makes the non-age-adjusted decline in heart disease deaths since the 1950s so remarkable.

This adjustment becomes important when considering statistics like cancer mortality. In 1950, unadjusted mortality for all cancers was 139.8 deaths per 100,000 people, rising to 188.7 in 2005. However, adjusting for the higher proportion of older people in the population, the same statistic becomes 193.9 in 1950, falling to 183.8 in 2005. *Health, United States, 2008* reports that the overall death rate for cancer fell by 15% between 1990 and 2005. Likewise, while a larger and older population means a higher raw incidence of cancer, in adjusted terms cancer incidence in the US actually fell from 475.4 cases per 100,000 people in 1990 to 442.7 in 2005. That is, despite more obesity, fewer people are getting cancer.

Health, United States, 2008 presents a complex and multi-layered picture. For example, I have neither highlighted some of the obvious and long-standing health disparities that exist in the United States, nor drilled down to statistics on specific health risk factors, such as the percentage of Americans with high total serum cholesterol, which has been declining since at least 1988, or the percentage with either diagnosed or undiagnosed diabetes, which increased from about 8% in 1988–1994 to 10% in 2003–2006. Nonetheless, when it comes to the increasing costs of the

United States health system, the document makes no mention of obesity, obesity-related disease or people's lifestyles. Instead, it states:

> The United States spends more on health per capita than any other country, and U.S. health spending continues to increase. Spending increases are due to increased intensity and cost of services, and a higher volume of services needed to treat an aging population.
>
> (National Center for Health Statistics 2009: 12)

England

It would be possible to read the 600 or so pages of *Health, United States, 2008* and completely fail to notice that an alleged obesity crisis exists. Brief references to body weight are sprinkled throughout the document, but the issue simply settles into the general scenery of American health. Excess body weight's role as a risk factor for some diseases is mentioned, but there is no sense that it requires the focused and urgent attention of the health community. The document even contains the heretical statement 'Research has found that persons who are overweight but not obese do not have excess mortality compared with persons of normal weight' (National Center for Health Statistics 2009: 32). I have seen this claim draw howls of derision and protest from mainstream obesity researchers at academic conferences. This is hardly surprising since, if it were true, it would go a long way to dismantling the edifice of obesity epidemic rhetoric, which has always relied on obscuring the difference between overweight and obesity.

But while the obesity epidemic has been a big story all over the Western world for at least a decade, there are differences in the way it has permeated popular and official discourse in different countries. In contrast to the previous American example, *Health Profile of England* singles out 'Reducing obesity and improving diet and nutrition' as one its six health priority areas (Department of Health 2006: 2). It concedes that large gains have been made in health but stresses the challenges that still exist. As well as reducing obesity, the six priority areas are: addressing health inequalities, smoking, sexual health, alcohol usage and mental health. With the possible exception of mental health, what we seem to have here is a particularly social view of health that prioritises personal behaviour and the influences on behaviour. In fact, *Health Profile of England* has almost nothing to say about individual diseases or families of disease, the performance of the nation's hospitals, doctors and health workers (things that get a great deal of attention in *Health, United States, 2008*) or medical science and research.

None of this is to suggest that the English government is less concerned about medical research or the practice of medicine generally. What is at stake here is more a question of how snapshots of particular nation's health are constructed. In the case of *Health Profile of England*, health seems to be synonymous with what many people would understand as the sphere of public health, focused on the so-called 'determinants' of health (such as inequality, lifestyle and others) rather than specific diseases and treatments. Once again, it is not that public health issues are ignored in *Health, United States, 2008*, but rather that they form only a small part of the overall picture.

It is almost as if the authors of *Health Profile of England* are saying to readers 'We all know what health is; it is not smoking, not having unsafe sex, not drinking, eating the right amount of good food and getting enough exercise'. As a result, no effort is made to explain why overweight or obesity are bad or to qualify or quantify the risks of having a BMI above 30. In fact, the document offers only two sentences in terms of justifying its focus on obesity. We must reduce obesity and improve diet and nutrition because:

> ... the rapid increase in child and adult obesity over the past decade is storing up very serious health problems for the future if it is not addressed effectively now. Effective action on diet and exercise now will help to tackle future heart disease, cancer, diabetes, stroke, high blood pressure, high cholesterol and a range of factors critical to our health.
>
> (Department of Health 2006: 15)

Unlike our American example, *Health Profile of England* makes inconsistent distinctions between overweight and obesity, sometimes quoting statistics for obesity alone but then in other places talking about overweight and obesity together. And while *Health, United States* uses the word 'epidemic' only in connection with influenza and AIDS, *Health Profile England* only uses it when talking about childhood obesity.

It is also noticeable that *Health Profile of England* devotes very little space to the health gains that have been made and makes no attempt to explain them. In fact, while mention is made of falling mortality rates for CVD and cancer generally, whether the incidences of these diseases are also decreasing is buried in the document's tables and draws no comment elsewhere except to say that the 'picture is mixed' (Department of Health 2006: 66) for cancer incidence. Overall, it appears that the incidence for all cancers (except non-melanoma skin cancers) is falling for men but rising for women. And while we might see the well-known large reductions in heart disease incidence and mortality in England as one of the great ongoing success stories of modern public health, incidence of heart disease is not mentioned in the text of the document at all and it occupies a single line in one of the document's many tables.

Like all the reports discussed in this chapter, *Health Profile of England* presents information on a wide range of topics and it would be wrong to suggest that it elevates obesity far above other concerns, such as alcohol abuse and sexual and mental health. However, it is consistent, I think, with a number of other signs that the English public health community is inclined to fight the war on obesity with particular zeal. For example, I was very much taken aback by a recent advertisement from the English government-supported 'Change4Life' campaign. The advertisement shows a photograph of an apparently healthy and happy female child holding a small cake alongside the words 'Is a premature death so tempting?'. The words are in large block white letters except for the word 'death', which is black. Below the image we read:

If current trends continue, nine out of ten children will grow up to have unhealthy amounts of fat in their bodies, a **government report** has concluded. So even if your kids look healthy today, adulthood could bring an early death from heart disease, Type 2 diabetes or cancer.

(4yourkids.org.uk, bold in original)

A second similar advertisement shows a young and apparently 'normal weight' boy holding the controls of a computer video game. The accompanying text is 'Risk an early death, just do nothing' (4yourkids.org.uk). Once again, 'death' is highlighted in inky blackness. These images are part of a wider Change4Life campaign that includes television advertisements and appears committed to emphasising the alleged link between childhood obesity and early death.

Compared with other Western countries, my anecdotal sense is that the tenor of English public health discourse is comparatively aggressive and uncompromising when it comes to obesity. Despite enjoying, by international standards, middle-of-the-road rates of overweight and obesity, England appears to have chosen a hot rather than cold war with its recalcitrant citizens.

New Zealand

The Executive Summary from *A Portrait of Health: Key Results of the 2006/07 New Zealand Health Survey* (Ministry of Health 2008) begins with 'Key findings' for adult and child health. In both areas, the executive summary leads with statements about how New Zealanders themselves rate their own health, perhaps establishing a glass-half-full rather than glass-half-empty orientation:

Overall, three out of five adults (60.6%) rated their own health as excellent or very good. European/Other men and women were more likely to report that their health was excellent or very good compared to all men and women in the population.

(Ministry of Health 2008: ix)

Overall, nine out of ten (87.2%) parents rated their child's health as excellent or very good.

(Ministry of Health 2008: xii)

Key findings are presented as a series of headings with a brief comment for each. It is not immediately clear how to interpret the order in which they appear, but the 'Key findings' for adults list begins with 'Use of primary health care services' and 'Public hospital use' and goes on to list ten others. 'Body size' is last in this list of twelve and is also last of nine 'Key findings for child health'.

The authors of *A Portrait of Health* do not use the term 'obesity epidemic', reserving 'epidemic' for their discussion of wintertime influenza. Nonetheless, the document's first substantive chapter, 'Health Behaviours and Risk Factors', devotes considerable space to behaviours that would conventionally be thought to play a role in body weight, such as 'fizzy drink intake', 'fast food intake', 'television watching' and 'active transport to school'. These sit amongst other sections on 'physical punishment by the primary caregiver', 'second-hand smoke' and 'problem gambling'. The substantial section titled 'body size' makes no predictions about the future and, as we saw in Chapter 3, concedes that obesity rates have slowed in recent years. This is in contrast with *Health Profile of England*, which emphasises a deteriorating body weight picture and warns of the consequences if the situation goes unchecked.

While *A Portrait of Health* includes standard statements about the association between increased body weight and risk for certain diseases, information is presented with studied neutrality, devoid of any sense that obesity is something anyone should be especially concerned about. Body size emerges here as one amongst many other health risks. In fact, the closest we get to alarm occurs when the obesity prevalence disparities across ethnic groupings are highlighted. Interestingly, though, while ten years worth of no change in obesity prevalence amongst adult New Zealanders might seem cause for celebration, this finding is left till last and draws no evaluative comment.

The next two chapters of *A Portrait of Health* contain information about the prevalence of a range of health conditions and the general health of New Zealanders. There is not a great deal of longitudinal data on which to draw, but that which does exist suggests mostly stable or improving trajectories. Between 2002–2003 and 2006–2007 there was a decrease in age-adjusted prevalence of arthritis, no change in stroke prevalence and no change in dental health amongst children. Between 1996–1997 and 2006–2007 there was no change in diabetes prevalence.

For general health status, approximately 90% of adult New Zealanders report that their health is 'good', 'very good' or 'excellent'. This appears to have changed little between 1996–1997 and 2006–2007. However:

> Between 2002/03 and 2006/07 there was a small but significant increase in the proportion of women who rated their health as excellent or very good, adjusted for age. Looking at Māori specifically, between 1996/97 and 2006/07 there was no change in the proportion of men and women reporting excellent or very good health, adjusted for age.
>
> (Ministry of Health 2008: 189)

It is true, of course, that documents of this kind have a lot of ground to cover in trying to summarise an entire nation's health. It is also true that the data presented here, much of it self-reported, could fail to pick up a looming but as yet unrealised crisis of chronic disease. It is perfectly possible for a range of reasons that *A Portrait of Health* has simply failed to describe the 'real' picture of New Zealand health, not noticing the obesity time-bomb ticking quietly before it explodes. Perhaps authorities were inclined to put a positive spin on health for political reasons. Whatever the explanation, if body weight is a particular and pressing health problem for New Zealand, this is not reflected in *A Portrait of Health*.

Australia

According to *Australia's Health 2008* (Australian Institute of Health and Welfare 2008), 'Australia's level of health continues to improve overall. Moreover, in most aspects of health Australia matches or leads other comparable countries' (6). In fact, Australian life expectancy has risen to rival many of the Western world's famously thin countries:

> In 2005, Australia's life expectancy at birth had risen to be one of the highest in the world. Life expectancy at age 65 for males ranked equal first with Japan, and for females it was equal second with France. Between the years compared, Australia's ranking among OECD countries improved markedly for mortality rates from coronary heart diseases, stroke, lung and colon cancer, and transport accidents, and in 2005 we had the lowest death rates from accidental falls in the OECD.
>
> (Australian Institute of Health and Welfare 2008: 7)

And later:

> Despite diseases and injuries remaining large problems, the situation is improving on many fronts. For example, death rates continue to fall for cancers, cardiovascular disease, asthma, chronic lung disease and injury. This is partly because of fewer of these problems arising in the first place – or at least arising later in people's lives – and partly because of better survival when they do arise.
>
> (Australian Institute of Health and Welfare 2008: 175)

Australia's Health 2008 does not describe a country on the edge of a public health crisis, neither driven by body weight nor by any other health variable. The claim that there are 'fewer of these problems arising in the first place' obviously cuts against the idea that there is more disease around or any characterisation of Australia as less healthy than in the past.

This has all been achieved despite rising overweight and obesity over the last thirty years and being ranked the amongst the Western world's fattest countries: 'Although there has been a small improvement in Australia's ranking for adult obesity rates since 1987, Australia remains in the "worst third" of all OECD countries on this measure' (Australian Institute of Health and Welfare 2008: 7).

Like most Western countries, Australia has experienced large decreases in mortality due to CVD in recent decades, with rates now below what they were 100 years ago. *Australia's Health 2008* makes the claim – standard across the research literature – that this is due to a combination of better medical care and a lower incidence of CVD. For example, with respect to coronary heart disease (CHD), a major subset of CVD:

> CHD death rates have fallen rapidly since the 1970s. In the latest decade alone (1996–2005), the age-standardised CHD death rate declined by 43% in

males and 41% in females. These declines are due to both a reduction in heart attacks and better survival.

(Australian Institute of Health and Welfare 2008: 184)

The overall picture for cancer in Australia is somewhat different:

Cancer was the leading cause of the total burden of disease and injury in Australia in 2003, with four-fifths of this burden due to premature death. However, over the last decade, improvements in early detection and treatment have resulted in improved survival and a clear decline in mortality for most cancers, despite the overall cancer incidence rate remaining virtually unchanged . . . It is projected that the number of new cases of cancer in 2008 will be around 108,000, a 10% increase on 2004. Most of the projected increase is because of growth in the population aged 60 years and over.

(Australian Institute of Health and Welfare 2008: 176–177)

While the obesity literature is full of claims about the connection between body weight and cancer, this relationship does not rate a mention in the report's 610 pages. And while there was a slight jump in cancer incidence between the mid-1980s and the mid-1990s, this is almost entirely explained by changing rates of skin cancer.

Rates of diabetes in Australia have risen significantly since the 1980s. The disease affected a little less than 1.5% of the age-adjusted population in 1989–1990 and just over 3% in 2004–2005. However, the extent to which this change is being driven by increased body weight is not known:

The prevalence of diagnosed diabetes in Australia based on self-reported information has more than doubled since 1989–90. Although an increase in the incidence of diabetes may play a major role in trends in diabetes prevalence, rising awareness in the community, better detection and better survival may also help explain them.

(Australian Institute of Health and Welfare 2008: 194)

Diabetes mortality is virtually unchanged since at least 1980.

Australia's Health 2008 also shows that while many obesity experts think Australians are getting sicker, this is not reflected in the small amount of data concerning what Australians say about themselves. The percentage of Australians who describe their health as 'good', 'very good' or 'excellent' has changed little since the mid-1990s, standing at 82.8% in 1995 and 84.3% ten years later.

As we saw in Chapter 2, outspoken obesity experts Paul Zimmet and Garry Jennings have repeatedly described obesity as 'our greatest public health concern'. There are few signs that this is a view shared by the authors of *Australia's Health 2008*. Although overweight and obesity are mentioned regularly throughout the document and highlighted in its concluding remarks, body weight contributes to a mixed general health outlook rather than standing out as a clear and pressing priority:

> The overview that emerges shows that health status is steady or improving and few of its indicators show unfavourable trends. Mortality especially is reducing and the levels of certain illnesses and diseases have reduced. Determinants of health show a more mixed picture with smoking-related indicators having improved levels, but rates of overweight and obesity increasing.
>
> (Australian Institute of Health and Welfare 2008: 476)

Dogs and monsters

It would clearly be wrong to claim that recent national health reports like the ones discussed in this chapter speak with one voice. Despite the global ubiquity of obesity epidemic rhetoric, health authorities in different countries have reacted in contrasting ways. Nonetheless, the modest proposal I offer here is that the obesity epidemic changes size and shape depending on where one stands to view it. Up close, in the journal and media comments of obesity experts, it looks like a monster on the verge of devouring us all. But a step or two further back, with a more holistic and complex perspective on health, obesity can morph into not so much a monster, but perhaps the public health equivalent of next door's barking dog, undeniably annoying but something much less than a catastrophe.

There will be some readers who will see this as an unimportant distinction. The argument often put to me is that it matters little whether we see obesity as a problem or a catastrophe, the main point being that we get on and do something about it. In the remainder of this book I will attempt to demonstrate why this is a mistaken point of view. In Chapters 6 and 7 I will show how crisis rhetoric has created a rhetorical backlash, most obviously embodied by the emergence of what I will call 'obesity scepticism'.

More immediately, though, in Chapter 5 Carolyn Vander Schee and I attempt to provide a series of examples of how crisis rhetoric can lead to patently misguided and ineffective policy responses. In other words, our argument will be that how an issue is framed does matter. The kinds of solutions we employ to solve any problem will always be, at least in part, a product of the kind of problem we think we are facing. A 'crisis' seems to demand that we do something, anything, as quickly as possible. And this is exactly the kind of policy environment the idea of an obesity epidemic has encouraged.

5 The obvious solution

With Carolyn Vander Schee

The world of obesity policy deserves a book of its own, although we hasten to add that this is not because there is a remarkable success story to tell. Anybody familiar with the area will know that the question of making an intentional and measurable impact on the body weight of large numbers of people is a long-standing policy dilemma (see Swinburn 2008 for a discussion).

When obesity researchers talk about what to do about the obesity epidemic they tend to use a small set of recycled phrases and ideas similar to the ones discussed in Chapter 2. For example, well aware of how few answers the research literature has produced, many offer some variation on the idea that we must act on the best available evidence as opposed to the best possible evidence. In other words, the situation is so serious that we cannot afford to wait until we have better answers to 'What works?'. This means that a wide range of policy responses, almost all of which have virtually no empirical record of efficacy, is suggested. Many are pursued with admirable zeal despite having little more than common-sense appeal to recommend them. Some have even been implemented in particular jurisdictions in various Western countries. For example, restrictions on food advertising during children's television hours, restaurant menus showing nutrient breakdowns and food labelling in supermarkets are or have been law at least somewhere in the world. In each case, advocates for these policies have essentially argued that these measures were at least worth a try, whatever the existing evidence did or did not say.

In this context, it is perhaps understandable why so many obesity researchers see schools as the obvious place to fight obesity. The academic literature is full of common-sense assertions about the need to start young, the amount of time children spend in schools and the relative capacity of governments to mandate policies with immediate effect in schools compared to other spheres of life (for a recent example, see Loeb 2009). In part, this chapter interrogates the common-sense appeal of schools as a frontline in the war on obesity. We do this by looking at the development of anti-obesity policy in one Western country, the United States. On one level, we show how misguided and naive the call to fight obesity through schools was and remains. On a deeper level, though, we want to use the focus on schools to draw wider conclusions about the global war on obesity. In other words, a focus on schools not only helps us to assess the likely success of school-based policies. The very fact that so many people think schools are an appropriate weapon also tells us something very interesting about the war itself.

Fighting obesity is not just something people feel very strongly about; it is also big business. Many people and organisations are now personally, emotionally and financially invested in the belief that fighting obesity as vigorously as possible is the right thing to do. Inevitably, this means that any attempt to interrogate the current policy environment will be met with hostility, confusion and misunderstanding. So, with a view to precision, it is worth at least trying to be completely clear about what is and is not the purpose of this chapter.

We have been watching and studying the war on obesity for long enough to know that sometimes good policies have negative side effects and that the reverse is also true; dubious policies and interventions can have unexpected benefits. There is little room for ideological purity here and we want to de-emphasise the sense that this chapter is an attempt to pass definitive judgments. We will not attempt to hide our own views, but we do not think that it is crucial that readers agree with us.

More important is what we take to be the most valuable contribution that researchers and scholars can make: to ask careful and informed questions about things that people take for granted. So, are schools really the right place to fight obesity? Are we sure that time and money is not being wasted? Are we sure that more good than harm is being done? More controversially, are the policies and interventions that we are see actually designed to fight obesity or simply create the impression of action? What plausible claims can be made about the successes and failures of these policies and interventions?

The war on obesity has generated a great deal of enthusiasm and energy to act and intervene; people want to do *something*. This is one of the predictable effects of calling obesity a 'crisis'. However, the argument we want to make is that this enthusiasm, coupled with the widely accepted lack of clear solutions, has created a complex and unpredictable policy dynamic. As a result, a great deal of time, money and energy has been expended with many obvious consequences but very little sign that obesity levels are likely to be affected. In part, this is because it is doubtful whether some anti-obesity policies and interventions were ever intended to do anything about obesity. Furthermore, many policies and interventions have been based on dubious assumptions about body weight, weight loss and behaviour change.

More important though, we want to argue that a policy environment that expends so much misguided and ill-informed energy is likely, very soon, to exhaust itself. This is particularly so if and where policy requires people to do things that seem pointless, tokenistic, unfair or counter-productive.

What doesn't work?

One of the challenges of trying to assess obesity policy is that many of the suggested solutions enjoy a level of common-sense appeal. For example, policies that attempt to increase the physical activity that children must do at school or mandate how much formal physical education they receive probably strike some people as sensible, low-risk and potentially effective courses of action. The trouble with common-sense solutions appears quickly enough, though, when we examine their built-in assumptions.

This last point is fundamental to understanding what follows in this chapter. We are not suggesting that there are cast-iron 'dos' and 'don'ts' when it comes to anti-obesity policy and we do not claim to have a crystal ball in which we can see the future impact of current policies. At the same time, for all our scepticism of much obesity research, we do think it offers us certain insights that should at least inform our actions. These insights will not hold in all contexts and at all times, but they do deserve to be factored into the thinking of people who really do want to wage war on obesity.

First, one of most obvious and yet regularly overlooked findings of obesity research is that losing weight is not difficult. Even substantial weight loss is common in the literature and methods for achieving this are quite well understood. However, weight loss that is sustained over the longer term is much rarer and it is this, not weight loss per se, that remains extremely challenging. It is this difficulty that underpins the widely reported poor success rate of diets: almost all diets can result in weight loss but almost none appear to work for very long. In turn, this is most likely not because most diets cease working, but because people find adhering to them difficult.

Second, school-based obesity interventions have a long and virtually unbroken record of failure in affecting children's body weight. This applies equally to interventions focused on food as well as physical activity. For example, Harrris, Kuramoto, Schulzer and Retallack's recently published a review of school-based physical activity interventions as far back as 1966:

> Our meta-analysis indicated that school-based physical activity interventions did not improve BMI. Therefore, such interventions are unlikely to have a significant effect on the increasing prevalence of childhood obesity. Our inferences appeared consistent among the many secondary analyses that we performed. Variation in the duration, intensity and structure of school-based physical activity interventions had minimal effects on short-term or long-term BMI change. The consistency of the BMI results among the studies included in the meta-analysis was striking ($r = 0.97$). This finding is important for policy-makers who continue to promote schoolbased physical activity as a central component of the strategy to reduce childhood obesity.
>
> (2009: 723)

People writing in this area also frequently mention two of the largest and most well-co-ordinated school intervention studies (Nader et al. 1999; Caballero et al. 2003), both of which failed to make an impact on children's BMI. The obvious question to ask here is that if we do not get the desired effect from well-resourced programs such as these, lead by experts in the field and with a built-in commitment to follow-up, what expectations should we hold for more piecemeal and less well-funded or well-co-ordinated interventions?

The reasons for these kinds of findings are numerous. For a start, whatever interventions we might implement in schools, it is not possible to isolate children from all the other influences in their lives that might mitigate against the intervention. This is particularly significant for interventions that attempt to influence children's food choices. A great deal of school reform research also reminds us that schools are busy places and teachers typically already have their hands full. In fact, educational history describes a rainbow of experts who have tried to use schools to solve their pet problem. So often, though, they forgot that their cause could only ever be one of many causes that schools were being asked to address. The idea that schools can and should solve society's problems has become increasingly popular in recent years, to the point that the overloading of school curricula and the work of teachers is now an area of research in its own right. To state what would seem the obvious, without rigorous prior planning and quality control, substantial targeted resourcing and consistent monitoring and follow-up, all school interventions, not just those focused on obesity, struggle to achieve their desired impact.

Obesity researchers, like many other commentators, also tend to pin a lot of hope on school physical education. This is something of a puzzle. Many have measured the physical activity that happens in physical education classes and consistently found that children expend only a small amount of energy in them. There is no reason whatsoever for seeing physical education as a viable childhood weight management strategy, yet it appears consistently in both academic and popular discussion about childhood obesity. Trost, for example, has argued that 'School PE programs are uniquely situated to address the epidemic of obesity and sedentary behavior plaguing our youth worldwide' (2006: 183). In fact, Trost writes as if school teachers have so much time on their hands that, as well as everything else, they should turn themselves into personal trainers, epidemiologists and behavioural therapists:

> Physical education teachers need to become more familiar with the population-level monitoring and surveillance data related to children's exposure to daily PE and the amount of physical activity provided by the average lesson. They also need to become critical consumers of scientific information pertaining to youth and physical activity . . . Most of all, there is an urgent need for physical educators to know and understand health behavioural change theory (e.g. social cognitive theory) and how to plan, implement and evaluate theory-based strategies to promote physical activity behavior in school physical education.
>
> (2006: 184)

We cannot imagine that Trost's suggestions will sound like good news to school teachers already working hard to meet the demands of parents, administrators, governments and the general public. Notice also the way researchers writing in this area appear to think that everyone else should see fighting obesity as central to their work and that they need to be educated into sharing this view. Another striking, if not bizarre, example of this appears in Budd and Hayman's (2008) article 'Addressing the childhood obesity crisis: a call to action' in the *American Journal of Maternal Child Nursing*. The article is instructive because it shows how calling something a crisis can profoundly change the way people think about themselves and their work. Space does not allow us to list all the ways Budd and Hayman think nurses could fight obesity, but they include informing patients about the marketing tactics of food companies, organizing media campaigns, advocating for particular municipal zoning laws and telling schools what food they should and should not serve. Budd and Hayman think that nurses should never miss an opportunity in their working and non-working lives to work and advocate against fatness. Depressingly, they write: 'Adults and children should have their BMI measured and charted at every health care visit and should be informed about how BMI is used to assess excess weight' (Budd and Hayman 2008: 115). Welcome to the brave new war on obesity. And fighting obesity is not something with which nurses can choose or not choose to involve them-selves: 'Nurses have a professional and moral obligation to advocate for social changes that promote healthy lifestyles, particularly for vulnerable populations such as children, the disabled, and persons living in poverty' (Budd and Hayman 2008: 117).

Returning to schools, there is another set of issues related to the general idea of using physical activity to manage children's weight. In this case, the common-sense observation that children will not much like boring, overly strenuous and unimaginative physical activity experiences is corroborated by research findings. Although admittedly an over-simplification, physical activity that the majority of children enjoy tends not to be the kind that results in weight reduction. To make matters worse for obesity warriors, there is little evidence that school-based physical activity programs help children to develop movement skill or even to increase their enjoyment of physical activity. And even if they did, physically active children do not automatically become physically active adults. Research tells us that as people move through their lives, their physical activity decisions and behaviours are driven as much by their immediate physical, economic and social circumstances as by previous habits and experiences.

To reiterate, we do not claim that any of this should silence further discussion about using schools to reduce obesity. While we remain sceptical, we also accept that researchers and advocates will want to keep trying to improve on past efforts by developing new strategies and techniques. We simply ask readers to keep these points in mind as we move now to consider policy in the United States and ask whether schools really are the obvious place to fight childhood obesity.

Simple or complex?

Obesity rhetoric constantly bounces between two extremes: on the one hand the idea that the problem is fiendishly complex and, on the other, the idea that it is blindingly simple. Public health experts often suggest that obesity 'has environmental, cultural, medical and social roots' that lack a 'single method for tackling the problem' (Albemarle State Policy Center 2009: 6). Others point out that obesity policy is:

> . . . weighed down by complexity, accentuated by the multi-level (global, European, national, regional and local) nature of modern systems of governance. It is also shrouded by ideological fears such as interventions being interpreted as 'nanny-ish' or restricting 'personal' choices in food and lifestyle.
>
> (Lang and Rayner 2007: 166)

However, when obesity politics are framed within the context of schools, these complexities seem to disappear. Consider Michelle Obama's recent statement regarding the school's role in tackling obesity. Calling obesity one of the 'greatest threats to America's health and economy' she told reporters:

> We don't need to wait for some new invention or discovery to make this happen. This doesn't require fancy tools or technologies. We have everything we need right now – we have the information, we have the ideas, and we have the desire to start solving America's childhood obesity problem . . . The only question is whether we have the will.
>
> (Hellmich 2010)

The idea that the problem is simple and the solutions are known is not necessarily played out in the realm of legislative politics. If it were simple we might expect to see anti-obesity policies passing legislatures with relative ease. Significant governmental effort has certainly gone into crafting school-based anti-obesity policies, yet legislating remains a highly contentious activity and there is still widespread disagreement about what to do. For example, in the United States, between January and October 2008 '. . . only 34 of the 320 bills related to obesity prevention were enacted into law, and only 15 of the 39 state legislatures that introduced or acted on legislation passed measures' (Albemarle State Policy Center 2009: 5). So, while a significant amount of legislation has been passed, this is partly because a huge amount has been proposed.

Even the state of Mississippi, a self-proclaimed leader in ratifying school-based anti-obesity laws, has experienced difficultly passing legislation. For example, in 2009, Democratic Mississippi Representative Omeria Scott proposed House Bill (HB) 1262. This act would have required the State Board of Education to mandate local school districts to provide low-fat snacks and meals to children identified by a physician as overweight. The bill died in committee. Representative Scott also proposed HB 791, which would have required school districts to collect annual BMIs on children in kindergarten and even-numbered grades up to tenth grade. This bill was also not endorsed. Another unsuccessful bill (HB 713), proposed by Democratic Representative Blain Eaton, would have amended the Healthy Students Act by permitting marching band participation to satisfy the physical education graduation requirement.

Putting to one side the question of whether state legislators should expend time and energy debating the merits of marching band calisthenics (see below for more detailed discussion of this issue), anti-obesity legislation in the United States is anything but a *fait accompli* despite the alleged urgency and simplicity of the situation. In addition, much of the legislation that is passed tends to be either weak or even purely symbolic. Even if there were a strong empirical case for them, there is currently little evidence that aggressive school-based policies are likely to pass into legislation.

The influence of corporate lobbies and special interest groups is one reason why ratifying tough school-based anti-obesity legislation is challenging. The recent agreement forged by the Alliance for a Healthier Generation (a joint initiative of the Clinton Foundation and the American Heart Association) as well as industry representatives from Cadbury-Schweppes, Coca-Cola, PepsiCo and the American Beverage Association illustrates this point well. In May 2006 representatives from the beverage industry announced that over a four-year period they would begin eliminating sodas from schools. More specifically, elementary and middle school students would be limited to purchasing bottled water, low-fat and non-fat milk and 100% fruit juice in eight- and ten-ounce servings respectively. High school students would have access to twelve-ounce servings and be permitted to purchase low-calorie juice drinks, sports drinks and diet sodas. By and large, the media praised the effort, applauding the soft drink industry's attempt to prioritise public health over corporate profits. Mr Clinton told the media that he believed that it was a 'truly significant thing for an industry to do, not entirely free of risks on their part' (Newman 2006). Subsequently, Governor of Arkansas Mike Huckabee, who was highly involved in anti-obesity initiatives in his state, told the media that he believed the companies made the agreement 'because they understand and accept the data about the trends, and they care about the future of our young people' (Newman 2006). Receiving less attention, however, were others who criticized the move, suggesting it was strategic and only negotiated to secure their interests. These critics argued that the soda industry was facing large and imminent lawsuits from a coalition of lawyers (the same group who successfully sued the tobacco industry) and the Center for Science in the Public Interest. The lawsuit was dropped as a result of this agreement. Importantly and somewhat characteristic of these kinds of concocted corporate self-imposed embargos, the agreement is voluntary and its success is entirely dependent on whether a school is willing to renegotiate their existing soda contracts. In essence, all the agreement does is allow schools, if they so choose, to default on a portion of their beverage contract (Burros and Warner 2006).

Attempts to reform the National School Lunch Program (NSLP) provide another interesting case in point. Introduced in 1946, today the NSLP serves one or more meals to more than 60% of children aged five to eighteen years at least once a week. Additionally, more than 60% of these meals are provided to children from low-income families at free or reduced cost (Ralston, Newman, Clauson, Guthrie and Buzby 2008). At the federal level, the Food and Nutrition Service, a branch of the United States Department of Agriculture (USDA), oversees the regulation of the program. For many years this agency has come under significant criticism, from their failure to adequately fund the program, their lax regulatory oversight and their over-reliance on unhealthy farm commodity foods to their concession-making with corporate entities.

Much of the trouble began in 1972, when Congress capitulated to pressure from industry lobbies to amend prior legislation (Pub. L. No. 91–248) which authorized the USDA to regulate the sale of foods sold outside the NSLP, otherwise known as 'competitive foods'. Competitive foods are all those foods sold in vending machines as well as *à la carte* items that are sold in the cafeteria. These foods are typically high in calories and fat, but they can tremendously increase a school's profit margin. The 1972 legislation allowed schools to sell competitive foods on the condition that the proceeds supported school organizations. Congress also appointed local and state agencies to oversee the sale of competitive foods, effectively alleviating the USDA, with its more stringent governance of the issue, from responsibility.

Then, in the early 1980s, the federal government drastically reduced funding for the NSLP. Fiscal restrictions sent an explicit message to state and local food authorities to find alternative ways to operate the NSLP independent of full federal support. Funding reductions, as well as the new statutory and regulatory leniency gave an open invitation for private companies to enter the very lucrative market of school food services (see Vander Schee 2004). Since this time, and more recently justified on the basis of the obesity epidemic, there have been numerous failed attempts to restore the USDA's regulatory authority in an effort to improve the nutritional content of food sold in schools. During the most recent reauthorization of NSLP, the debate over vending machines came into full play. According to Haskins, while there was bipartisan agreement that the reauthorization should address vending machines in schools, there was a divergence of opinions about what Congress should do:

> Democrats wanted to exert federal control over vending machines by giving the Secretary of Agriculture authority over all food available in schools rather than just school lunch and breakfast. Giving such authority to the secretary was expected to result in the removal, alteration in content, or restriction of operating hours for vending machines . . . Republicans wanted local authorities to figure out their own solutions.

> (2005: 17)

In the end, unable to reach consensus and bowing to pressure from the food and beverage industry, Congress decided to leave vending machines in schools but require schools to develop 'wellness policies' (P.L. 108–265), where schools would outline their 'goals for nutrition education and physical activity as well as provide guidelines for all food sold in the schools' (Haskins 2005: 17). To ensure that schools would comply, Congress used federal contributions to the NSLP and Child Nutrition Act of 1966 (42 U.S.C. 1771 et seq) as a kind of surety. There is nothing particularly new about the federal government relinquishing direct control over the finer details of policy and passing this responsibility to state and local governments. However, because they presumably want to ensure that states and local governments take this responsibility seriously, they often levy their financial influence, enacting something of a carrot-stick approach to policy-making.

Thus in 2004, Congress passed the Child Nutrition and WIC Reauthorization Act of 2004 that outlined their Wellness Policy mandate. This gave schools till the end of the 2006 school year to comply with the stipulations of the legislation. By and large, the legislation placed the responsibility of developing wellness policies at the local level. This was done strategically, of course, based on the premise that the individual needs of each district could be better addressed at the local level. According to the new federal requirements, local entities were to set goals and establish regulations for nutrition education, physical activity, campus food provision and other school-based activities for the purpose of promoting student wellness. Additionally, local districts were required to involve a broad group of individuals in policy development and to have a plan for measuring policy implementation. The recent flurry of school-based health policies, then, is a direct consequence of the Wellness Policy legislation. Additionally, following the federal mandate, a number of state governments established specific guidelines as well as minimum criteria that local districts must follow when crafting their wellness policies.

For individual schools, meeting the terms and conditions of the new federal and state mandates can represent something of a compliance nightmare. To help ease the burden and to assist schools, a number of states have created entirely new organisational entities. Mississippi's Healthy Students Act (SB 2369) provides an interesting case in point. Signed into law by Republican Governor Haley Barbour during the 2007 legislative session, the act is perhaps the most comprehensive form of school-based anti-obesity legislation seen anywhere in the country. Following the bill's ratification, it was widely praised in state and national media outlets as a positive and progressive development in anti-obesity policy. News articles reporting on the legislation went so far as to call Mississippi a 'national leader' (Byrd 2009). Among other items, the bill establishes some of the most stringent standards for physical and health education set anywhere in the country. Not only do these requirements outline a minimum number of instructional minutes per week for each grade level, but at the high school level these specifications are tied to graduation. The bill also explicitly defines what qualifies as adequate physical activity. In terms of school-based nutrition, districts are legislated to act in accordance with new state standards on the following issues: what constitutes a healthy food and beverage, methods of food preparation, marketing food to students and staff, food preparation ingredients and products, minimum and maximum time allotments for students and staff lunch and breakfast periods and the availability of food items during the lunch and breakfast periods of the Child Nutrition School Breakfast and Lunch Programs.

While the Healthy Students Act (SB 2369) attempts to govern a greater number of issues (from curricular decisions to food preparation), it also significantly increases the number of individuals required to participate in the policy process. For example, the legislation requires the state to hire a 'Physical Education Coordinator'. The bill not only specifies the precise qualifications the Coordinator must possess, but it also stipulates those groups who are required to be involved in the selection process. Before a state Physical Education Coordinator can be hired, the following groups must be consulted: the Governor's Commission on Physical Fitness and Sports; the Mississippi Council on Obesity Prevention and Management; the Task Force on Heart Disease and Stroke Prevention; the Mississippi Alliance for Health, Physical Education, Recreation and Dance; and the Mississippi Alliance for School Health.

At the local level, we see a similar trend. The local school board is instructed to appoint members to the local school health council, ensuring that an individual from each of the following groups is represented: parents who are not employed by the school district, the director of local school food services, teachers, administrators, district students, health care professionals, the business community, law enforcement, senior citizens, the clergy, non-profit health organizations and faith-based organisations. One of the primary functions of the local school health council is to recommend appropriate practices on issues related to health education, physical education, nutritional services, parental/community involvement, instruction to prevent the use of tobacco, drugs and alcohol, physical activity, health services, healthy environment, counselling and psychological services, healthy lifestyles, and staff wellness. On all these matters, local health councils are told that they may 'adopt rules and regulations that may be more stringent but not in conflict with those adopted by the State Board of Education' (Mississippi Legislature 2007). Thus, not only are school leaders required to comply with the new regulations governing the process of policy-making, they also have to navigate the new policy terrain created by this highly complex process.

For all its good intentions, Mississippi's attempt to create an inclusive environment for policy-making is complex and bureaucratic. On the surface, what Mississippi seems to have ended up with is a policy response designed to avoid direct conflict with the food corporations – at least at the federal level – and shift the heavy burden of policy enactment to the local level. Given our earlier points about the lack of success schools have had in this area, what confidence could we have that the end product of this long and winding policy process will produce successful body weight management strategies? Additionally, do all schools have the organisational capacity, expertise and resources needed to carry out this unfunded mandate? In Mississippi, for example, in an effort to assist schools deal with the new federal and state legislation, the state created the Office of Healthy Schools (a branch of the Mississippi Department of Education) to provide technical assistance and services to schools. In 2008, the Office of Healthy Schools hosted the Mississippi Healthy Students Act Institute, a multi-day seminar designed to assist school leaders face their new responsibilities and obligations under the requirements of the Act. Another important issue is whether all those required to serve on Mississippi's local health council, including parents, the business community, law enforcement officers, senior citizens and members of the clergy, have adequate expertise in epidemiological or public health or sufficient administrative knowledge of the logistics of school-based affairs to design effective policies. Is what we have here a structure designed to fight obesity or simply avoid offending the sensibilities of certain stakeholder groups?

While Mississippi's legislative response to the federal mandate is certainly intriguing, its experience in crafting and implementing anti-obesity policies is not unique. In the following sections, we examine the ways in which schools across the country have addressed the obesity issue in response to the federal Local Wellness Policy legislation or state mandates or, in other cases, simply as a result of individual school initiatives.

Anti-obesity policies and school employees

When the 'war on obesity' becomes central to a school's purpose and mission, as it has for many schools, the patchwork quilt of policies often has far-reaching effects. One dimension of their influence, and one that garners relatively little attention, is the way in which these policies affect teachers' work. In some cases the new mandates and resulting policies explicitly alter the job requirements and expectations of those employed at the school, such as teachers having to inspect the nutritional content of student lunches brought from home. In other cases, the influence of these policies may be experienced more subtly so that almost everyone, from student to custodian, becomes implicated, responsible or tangentially involved.

Perhaps the most dominant message articulated in media and policy discourses pertaining to school leaders' obesity-related responsibilities centres on their designation as healthy lifestyle role models. For example, according to the World Health Organization,

> Health promotion for school personnel is important because teachers and other staff need to be aware of and responsible for the messages they give as role models to students and others. Furthermore, evidence suggests that promoting the health of school staff by encouraging physical activity and healthy diet may improve staff productivity and mood, and reduce medical/ insurance expenses.
>
> (2008: 22)

In a similar vein, the Council of State Governments contends that schools should enact wellness programs for school staff as well as 'policies to enable staff to serve as role models and increase productivity' (Council of State Governments 2007: 31). Likewise, the National School Boards Association (NSBA) writes that 'school staff have the potential to be very powerful role models for students' (National School Boards Association 2000: E-15). It is interesting to consider the ways in which various schools take up these recommendations and articulate them into school policies and practices. In Minnesota, for example, districts disseminate the following survey to teachers. The questionnaire, entitled, 'Teachers – Are you a FitKid Role Model?' contains the following questions for teachers to answer:

1. Do your students see how active you are around the school?
2. Do you encourage your students to move at recess time?
3. Do you provide information to parents about safe recreation centers or after-school programs in your area?
4. Do your students see you eat nutritious foods?
5. Do your students see you drink milk or water instead of pop/coffee?
6. Do you serve nutritious foods in your classroom?
7. Do you refrain from talk about dieting in front of your students as well as likes and dislikes?
8. Do you encourage your students to eat school breakfast and lunch?
9. If you notice a student is hungry or comes to school without breakfast do you refer them to the breakfast or lunch program?
10. Do you help your child's school create a healthy school environment?
11. Do you incorporate nutrition messages into the curriculum you are teaching?
12. Do you eat school meals (breakfast and lunch)?

(Minnesota Department of Education 2008)

After completing the questionnaire, teachers are asked to create and commit to individual health goals corresponding to each of the twelve survey questions. If a teacher indicated that they did not serve nutritious food in their classroom, they are asked to create a goal to achieve this. What is more, they would be asked to record their commitment to achieving this goal. To assist teachers in realising their goals, they are directed to various school resources such as, 'Teachers as Lifestyle Role Models – Ideas to Help Your Students Lead Healthy Lifestyles' and 'Ideas to Help Your Children Lead Healthy Lifestyles'.

The notion that teachers have a responsibility to display certain behaviors and virtues is not a new phenomenon. There is a long historical tendency to hold teachers to higher standards both inside and outside schools. There are a few elements of this particular document, however, that make it a particularly instructive example. Perhaps the most fascinating aspect is that it seems less concerned about whether teachers actually accomplished particular health behaviours and more concerned about whether the students saw the teacher perform them or abstain from them.

In many ways, the suggestion that engaging in or abstaining from specific behaviours makes one a good role model blurs the distinction between notions of health and morality. If nothing else, it positions teachers, willingly or unwillingly, as a kind of public exemplar from which children will mimic upright or inappropriate behaviours. Performing health becomes a way to distinguish those who have learnt the virtues of self-regulation and self-discipline from those who have not. Simultaneously, the document works to create new ideas about the obligations and responsibilities of teachers to do their bit in the overall effort to reduce childhood obesity. It is also interesting that an important goal seems to be consistency of message. In order for students to learn how to be healthy they must be continually exposed to a series of congruent health messages. For teachers, this means that they must incorporate health into many aspects of their work. In this way, health becomes a kind of school-wide motif, influencing everything from a teacher's choice of beverage to the content of the curriculum.

Given the complexity of health behaviour change, we might also wonder about the assumption that children are so impressionable and their health behaviours so flexible that even witnessing a teacher might persuade them to act or not act accordingly. In fact, there is a strong sense in these kinds of policies that health as a concept is being dumbed down into a simple and easily definable enterprise. Neither teachers nor students are encouraged to engage in thoughtful reflection about their health. In fact, thinking about health, rather than blindly following a set of behaviours, would seem counter to the spirit of the war on obesity in schools, where conformity appears to be the primary virtue (see Gard 2008 for a discussion of this issue in the Canadian context).

All of this raises important questions about the normative expectations we hold for those who work at schools. What do we expect teachers to do, be or perform, and for what purposes? Certainly the above example reflects a kind of direct behavioural manipulation. However, we also see efforts directed at altering teachers' health status for the purpose of achieving various economic ends. While it would be naive and simplistic to suggest that straightforward distinctions exist between ideological and economic motivations, we can certainly see the influence of these in shaping policy.

Consider, for example, the growing trend to use financial incentives or disincentives to influence teachers' health behaviours. In Kansas, Unified School District 232 has mimicked a form of the NBC primetime show 'The Biggest Loser'. Participation in the program is voluntary and results are posted online under the banner 'Winning with Wellness.' Program participants also have a chance to earn 'wellness points' for engaging in particular health behaviours. Participants are told that the more wellness points they earn, the better their chances are of winning prizes (Unified School District #232 2010).

Across the country there is an increasing number of programs similar to the one in Kansas. And while most programs are voluntary and use participation incentives to motivate participants, they can still be seen as potentially problematic. On one hand, not all teachers will have the ability or resources needed to achieve the various performance targets. On the other hand, these programs tend to inspire a kind of negative collegial policing. Consider the wellness initiative at North Idaho College. Speaking about the drawbacks of the program, the Wellness Coordinator admitted that the program does not always enhance collegial camaraderie. For example, while grocery shopping he had to explain to a co-worker, 'that the corn dogs in his cart were not for him but his 17-year-old son' (Wilson 2009: A1). As with many similar initiatives, the participants in the program at North Idaho College can earn up to $2,000 a year toward medical expenses if they sign affidavits pledging that they will adhere to the program requirements.

Another issue relates to whether these programs will remain voluntary. For example, a number of state legislators, including those in Tennessee, West Virginia, Alabama and North Carolina, have entertained mandatory obesity penalties for state workers. In 2008 Alabama passed legislation mandating that all state workers receive a health screening. If a problem like high blood pressure, cholesterol, diabetes or obesity is found, state employees are given one year to join a wellness program, see a doctor or improve their health on their own to avoid a $300 per year insurance penalty (Alabama State Employees Insurance Board n.d.).

Needless to say, school employees are not always comfortable with school-based anti-obesity policies, particularly ones that directly encroach on individual liberties. In February 2009, a group of Oregonian teachers lobbied representatives to support House Bill 2419, which would counteract a 2007 law that restricted the sale of soda, fruit juices and high-calorie snack foods in schools. An unintended consequence of the law, however, was that it became illegal for teacher lounges to sell the banned food. While members of Oregon's Nutrition Policy Alliance urged legislators 'not to give in to the teachers' cravings,' teachers argued that the law treated them like children (Cole 2009). Siding with the teachers, representatives from Oregon's Education Association pointed out that a teacher's decision to 'buy a bag of peanuts or cookies' should not be cause for legislative concern (Cole 2009).

Anti-obesity policies and students

In terms of school food and nutrition, there is no compelling empirical evidence to direct policy action. This is similar to the situation for other policy targets, such as physical education, health education, fitness testing and BMI reporting. As a result, nutrition policies are subject to a range of personal, ideological, individual, financial and political forces. While this has always been the case in educational policy-making, food offers a particularly intriguing case. For example, the contradictory nature of various nutrition policies raises the question of whether they have more to do with the vested interests of those engaged in the process than in the efficacy of the policies themselves.

The issue of what food children should be permitted to consume at school has become central in the obesity policy debate. Here we are not even talking about typical vending machine regulations, but rather controversies about such things as what foods children are allowed to consume during classroom celebrations. Many districts, like Central Stickney School District #110 in Chicago, Illinois, have implemented entire moratoriums on popular celebratory food items. In this district the following letter was sent home to parents and guardians:

> Dear Parent/Guardian:
>
> Schools have a responsibility to help students establish lifelong habits of healthy eating patterns and regular physical activity. By establishing healthy habits early in life, children can dramatically reduce their health risks and increase their chances for longer, more productive lives. You love your children and you want the best for them. You can show this by creating opportunities for them to make healthy food choices. **Foods such as candy, cake, cupcakes, and ice cream do not meet dietary guidelines and will not be served to our children**.

The list of food and beverages below are consistent with the Dietary Guidelines for Americans.

HEALTHY SNACK LIST/SPECIAL OCCASIONS

* Raw vegetable sticks or slices with low fat dressing or yogurt dip
* Fresh fruit wedges-watermelon, cantaloupe, honeydew, pineapple, oranges, etc.
* Sliced fruit – apples, pears, peaches, plums, nectarines, etc.
* Dried fruits – raisins, cranberries, apples, apricots
* Single serving apple sauce
* Trail mix
* Pretzels or reduced fat crackers
* Goldfish or Wheat Thins
* Granola bars, graham crackers, fig bars
* Fat free or low fat pudding cups
* Bottled water

All of the items listed above are believed to be consistent with the intent of our school wellness policy to promote student health and reduce childhood obesity. We encourage all parents to use the above list as a guide in providing healthy snacks for our children. *Snacks which do not meet nutritional standards will NOT be served to students. Such items include, but are not limited to, cake, cupcakes, cookies, and candy.*

Sincerely,

Principal
                (Central Stickney School District #110 2009, formatting in original)

Not all schools support this kind of policy. In Enid, Oklahoma, for example, parents have been advised that, 'Yes. Cookies, candy and other goodies can be shared for classroom parties because they are special events. This teaches students that all foods can be enjoyed in moderation' (Enid Public Schools n.d.). A slight variation of this policy is found in Duval County, Florida, where the district leaves the decision to the discretion of the principal. In this county, the district's policy states that '. . . class parties are a tradition in public education. These parties may be held with the permission of the school principal, in moderation . . .' (Duval County Public Schools n.d.). Here, individual principals are left to decide whether sweet treats are eaten or prohibited.

These examples highlight what we think is one of the fundamental tensions in trying to use schools to fight obesity. Addressing an issue like permissible food by having a blanket rule for all schools is unlikely to be popular or effective. And yet, what sense does it make for schools to enact different and, in some cases, contradictory policies, particularly if what we are trying to do here is address a public health emergency? Rather than leading to clarity, this tension might instead give us pause to at least wonder whether having to generate, communicate and police these policies is not simply of a waste of educators' time and energy.

The debate around if, when and how often sweet treats can be enjoyed at school has even become a legislative affair, although not all constituents believe that schools should necessarily limit children's access to certain foods. A significant point of resistance has come from schools' Parent Teacher Associations (PTAs) because, as in many schools, PTAs often rely on bake sales and pizza days for fundraising. Under most of the new regulations these activities are no longer permissible, as foods sold for fundraising do not meet the more stringent nutritional requirements. Some schools have attempted to avoid these conflicts altogether by designing policies to satisfy PTAs. These schools place time and location restrictions on certain foods, effectively allowing PTAs to sell their food in designated locations and/or during specified times of the day. Schools that have not been amenable to PTA fundraising efforts often find themselves defending their policies against a well-co-ordinated attack. Consider, for example, the call to action that *PTO* [Parent Teacher Organization] *Today* posted on their website:

> If your group's activities have been limited by a wellness policy with food restrictions you think are too strict, set up a meeting with the appropriate administrator to talk about the situation. Emphasize the educational activities, tools, and programs made possible by parent group fundraising. Point out the community goodwill and parent involvement resulting from family events, many of which include popular refreshments like donuts and brownies.
>
> (Harac 2008)

PTAs are not the only groups complaining about new rules that restrict bake sales on school campuses. In New York, hundreds of angry students campaigned against the Department of Education's new policy that places limitations on the content and timing of students' bake sales. Not only did students argue that the 'new reform actually restricts the freedom of students' and 'creates a monopoly for companies that are contracted with the Department of Education', but it makes it very difficult for student groups to raise money (Phillips 2009). In New York schools, as in many schools across the country, bake sales are used to generate additional funds for student groups. New York students argued that many groups – everyone from the Ultimate Frisbee Club to the Literary Magazine Group – would be negatively affected by the ban.

Other groups have taken their plight a step further. When the state of Texas banned classroom celebrations involving sweet treats, parents and PTAs across the state protested vehemently. Likening cupcake bans to 'an assault on the national identity' (Schulte 2006), protestors successfully lobbied legislators to draft the 'Safe Cupcake Amendment'. Passed with bi-partisan support, the amendment exempts classroom celebrations involving cupcakes on a child's birthday from the state's school nutrition bill.

Some policies have gone as far as stipulating the exact amount of fat, calories, vitamins and minerals permissible for foods sold in schools. As it turns out, precision does not necessary guarantee a better policy. Mississippi's Office of Healthy Schools has generated a detailed list of prohibited and acceptable foods. Portion sizes of prohibited foods are also specified. Despite this precision there was confusion regarding one particular item: Frito Lay Baked Doritos, Nacho Cheese Flavor. This item appeared on both the approved as well as the denied list. More specifically, the 1-ounce bag was listed on the denied list and the 1 3/8-ounce bag was listed on the approved list. For a state implementing nutrition policies with the goal of reducing children's caloric intake, banning the small bag but approving the larger bag seems contradictory. Not so, at least according to the Office of Healthy Schools:

> The size of the package of the Frito-Lay Baked Doritos on the approved list is 1 3/8 oz. The size of the package of the Frito-Lay Baked Doritos on the Denied list is 1 oz. To meet the criteria for an accepted product include number of calories, % of calories from fat, total fat, saturated fat; the % of weight of the sugar and whether the product contains 5% of the RDV [Recommended Daily Value] for Fiber, Vit A, Vit C, Calcium, Iron, Vit D, Vit E, thiamine, niacin riboflavin, zinc; and 3 grams of protein. The smaller bag of baked Doritos meets all of the requirements except the 5% of the RDV and protein. Since the larger bag has more chips and therefore more nutrients, it meets all of the criteria including the 3 RDV and protein.
>
> (Office of Healthy Schools 2008)

Interestingly, legislated restrictions and bans on specific food items are becoming something of a trend for policy-makers. In Arkansas, for example, the following regulations apply to serving French fries to students:

> ELEMENTARY – French fries/fried potato products will be offered to elementary students NO MORE THAN ONCE PER WEEK. French fry (deep fat fried) serving size can be no more than three-fourths (3/4) cup by volume per serving.
>
> MIDDLE AND JUNIOR HIGH – French fries/fried potato products (deep fat fried) will be offered to middle and junior high school students in a serving size NO LARGER THAN one (1) cup by volume.
>
> HIGH SCHOOL – French fries/fried potato products (deep fat fried) will be offered to senior high students in a serving size NO LARGER THAN one and one-half (1½) cups by volume.
>
> (Arkansas Department of Education 2005)

While it is perhaps reasonable that schools might recommend different serving sizes for students based on their age, it does seem somewhat arbitrary to limit French fries to no more than once a week at the elementary level and then eliminate this ban at the middle school level. One might also wonder why schools are serving French fries at all, if they are considered unhealthy. Why once a week? Why not simply stop serving French fries entirely? The random nature of the French fry policy is similar to the current trend in vending machine politics. Many schools are reluctant to eliminate vending machines altogether because they are dependent on their profits, yet wanting to display a show of commitment to health, many schools stipulate that 50% of foods available in vending machines meet particular nutritional requirements. The other 50% of foods are not subject to these nutritional guidelines. Rules like this raise questions about the policy's ultimate purpose. If the goal of the policy is to limit children's access to unhealthy foods, how effective will the 50% rule be? Or is this an example of policy symbolism, where policies stand for an idea without doing very much to prosecute the idea?

Consider also the case of Massachusetts Fluffernutter Amendment. When Senator Jarrett Barrios discovered that his third grade son was served a Fluff (marshmallow spread) and peanut butter sandwich for lunch, the Senator drafted an amendment to alter the state's school nutrition bill by limiting schools from serving the marshmallow treat to only once a week. Barrios's amendment was met with immediate resistance from across the state. Newspapers ran commentary from angry protestors who called the move 'almost anti-American' and 'definitely anti-Massachusetts' (Calloway 2006). A local delicacy, Marshmallow Fluff is a popular New England food. In a counter-retaliatory move, State Representative Kathi-Anne Reinstein filed her own bill to make Fluffernutter the official state sandwich. In a letter drafted to gain the support of fellow House Representatives, Reinstein urged her colleagues to 'preserve the legacy of this local delicacy' and argued that Fluff 'contains no fat and is only one point in the Weight Watchers diet program' (Calloway 2006). Barrios eventually dropped his amendment, claiming that he simply drafted the legislation to make a point.

In recent years, school-based physical fitness testing mandates have become a popular policy initiative, purportedly with a view to motivate children to be more physically active. In 2007, eleven states enacted laws concerning mandatory student BMI measurement and/or physical fitness assessments (Albemarle State Policy Center 2008). In 2008, eleven states considered similar legislation and almost half of these bills were enacted (Albemarle State Policy Center 2009). With respect to fitness testing, the state of California provides an interesting example because the state has been conducting the tests for many years and a number of legislators are planning to mimic California's program in their own state. This begs the question of whether the California program is worth replicating.

California first began fitness testing students in 1976. However, the recent re-authorisation of the mandate under the 1995 California Assessment of Academic Achievement Act (Assembly Bill 265) is the legislation that has garnered the most publicity. In 1996, the state ratified Section 60800 of the bill, which created even greater accountability requirements and, further, required schools to use a standardised fitness test programme, FITNESSGRAM®, to record and monitor student fitness levels (California Department of Education 2009). Using the

FITNESSGRAM® programme, schools are told to assess students on six criteria: aerobic capacity, abdominal strength and endurance, upper body strength and endurance, body composition, trunk extensor strength and flexibility. According to the legislation, schools must administer the FITNESSGRAM® physical fitness test (PFT) to all students in grades five, seven and nine. The California State Department of Education (SDE) then collects the PFT scores and posts aggregate results on their website. Results are also passed along to the Governor and State Legislature. Additionally, individual schools are required to inform students of their personalized results and include school-wide summaries in their annual School Accountability Report Card (California Department of Education 2009).

According to the SDE, the primary goal of fitness testing is to 'assist students in establishing lifetime habits of regular physical activity' (California Department of Education 2009). The data obtained through testing, however, has a variety of uses. The state claims that students can use the information to 'assess and plan an individual fitness program'. Teachers can use the information to inspire curricular innovation and parents can use it to 'understand their children's fitness levels'. It can be also used to monitor and track student fitness levels for epidemiological purposes.

Aside from the more obvious questions about the additional time, resources, and personnel needed for schools to carry out this mandate, and in addition to the potential negative effects that this kind of high stakes standardized PFT has on students, there are issues pertaining to the mandate's highly problematic assumptions. For example, is it reasonable to assume that taking a fitness test on three occasions over a five-year time period will establish 'a lifetime habit of regular physical activity'? Do most fifth graders have the necessary knowledge, capacity and resources to 'assess and plan an individualized fitness program' based on their personalized PFT results? And, even if they do, how many children enjoy the necessary autonomy in their lives to carry this out?

Furthermore, is it reasonable to assume that the simple act of testing students motivates them to alter their physical activity behaviours? Mass numeracy and literacy testing of students happens around the world and there is no evidence that these tests help to 'motivate' students. Aside from these issues, we are also interested in the kinds of rhetorical effects that programs like this inspire. Consider California's State Superintendent of Instruction Jack O'Connell's press release commenting on the November 2009 results:

> I am pleased that our students continue to make strides toward becoming physically fit . . . The percentage of students who are in the healthy fitness zone is increasing. However, as a state we must continue to improve . . . Our students must take responsibility for their fitness, health, and overall well-being so they can compete on the playing field, in the classroom, and on the global stage.
>
> (California Department of Education, Communications Division 2009)

The curiosities in a statement like this are considerable. Perhaps most obvious is its emphasis on rugged self-reliance, individualism and competition. But there is surely also a comical edge here in the way O'Connell seems to imagine children doing a few extra abdominal crunches today and moving on to world domination tomorrow. We might also wonder how the publicly available FITNESSGRAM® data will be used to inform subsequent educational policies. Recently, researchers have begun correlating students' FITNESSGRAM® scores with their standardized test scores. University of California, Los Angeles researchers, for example, came to the following recommendation, following their examination of the data: 'Schools and parents seeking to optimize their students' academic performance should take heed . . . for optimal brain function, "it's good to be both aerobically fit and to have a healthy body shape"' (Hendry 2010). The researchers go on to argue that if these trends continue '. . . schools will have to reverse their recent disinvestment in physical education ostensibly for the purposes of boosting student achievement' (Hendry 2010).

What brand of physical education would emanate from recommendations like this? Discussing California schools' lacklustre 2008 results, Dr Harold Goldstein, Executive Director of the California Center for Public Health Advocacy, told the press that 'P.E. as it's taught today has little link to these fitness measures' (Knoll 2008). He went on to say that 'This is one of those things where you actually want kids to be taught for the test and it's not being done' (Knoll 2008). Goldstein's recommendation, then, is to better align physical education to the six FITNESSGRAM® criteria. This, he argues, would result in higher FITNESSGRAM® scores. In all of this a simple and consistent research finding is missed: children just do not like physical education programs that have the sole purpose of making them fitter. They much prefer to enjoy themselves.

Interestingly enough, the state of California is also endorsing the academic achievement/fitness connection. In a recent press release, the SDE announced that those students who won the Governor's Fitness Challenge Competition came from the state's highest academically performing schools. The Challenge is a pledge students make to be physically active for 30–60 minutes at least three times a week for a month. Winners of the Challenge share nearly $400,000 in physical activity equipment and cash rewards for their schools (California Department of Education, Communications Division 2009). Programs like this beg questions about the wisdom of further advantaging schools that are already excelling in this area.

Policies involving physical activity in schools are the subject of widespread debate. However, most policies, particularly those that necessitate a change to the existing environment, require additional resources such as time, energy, equipment and personnel to implement. One of the many questions pertaining to policy implementation often involves which governing body (at the federal, state or local level) will take responsibility for funding these new mandates. Very often, state and local entities criticise the federal government for ratifying legislation that is partly or entirely unfunded. In many of these under-funded or unfunded mandates, the federal government derives the benefit of widespread media applause for their concern and apparent commitment, while state and local governments are left to pick up the tab. One way to garner positive media attention without unduly antagonising state and local policy-makers is to create mandates that have high exchange value without requiring a significant modification to the existing environment.

A prime example of this is the Child Nutrition and WIC Reauthorization Act of 2004 (Public Law 108–265). It mandates that school districts participating in the NSLP or the Child Nutrition Act adopt a Local Wellness Policy. As previously mentioned, this legislation requires schools to create goals for nutrition, physical activity and other school-based activities designed to promote student wellness. Concerns about childhood obesity were used as a central justification for greater local governance and accountability in this area.

Over the past few years, this legislation, as well as the ways in which states have implemented it, has received a great deal of criticism, with a few recurring complaints. First, since the mandate was unfunded, schools have been left to independently finance their wellness endeavours – a situation that leads to some schools simply ignoring the legislation (see Dyson, Amis, Wright, Vardaman and Ferry forthcoming). In addition, as Chriqui points out, 'while the majority of school districts are following the letter of the law, they aren't really following the spirit of the law, because the majority of these policies lack teeth' (Robert Wood Johnson Foundation 2009). Chriqui goes on to suggest that Local Wellness Policies are 'fragmented, and they don't include provisions for monitoring, enforcing, or conducting ongoing review and revision of the policy' (Robert Wood Johnson Foundation 2009). These comments on the status of the law, as well as its dubious implementation measures, do not bode well for policies intended to encourage children to become more physically active.

In some cases, it appears that the language of legislation has been strategically chosen to give the impression of concern and action when, in fact, little (if any) change to the existing policy environment is actually mandated. Perhaps as a consequence of both ambiguous legislative language and such a wide variety of constituents participating in the policy-making process, there have been a number of heated debates focusing on the role of physical education and physical activity in schools.

One of the most interesting controversies regarding implementation of the Local Wellness Policy mandate has centred on the way the terms, 'physical education' and 'physical activity' are used within the legislation. While the term 'physical education' actually appears nowhere in the original mandate, schools are mandated to develop appropriate goals for physical activity. While some would see this as an insignificant distinction, these terms have distinct meanings and implications for administrators and educators alike. According to the National Association for Sport and Physical Education:

> School physical education programs offer the best opportunity to provide physical activity to all children and to teach them the skills and knowledge needed to establish and sustain an active lifestyle. Physical education teachers

assess student knowledge, motor and social skills, and provide instruction in a safe, supportive environment . . . Physical activity is bodily movement of any type and may include recreational, fitness and sport activities such as jumping rope, playing soccer, lifting weights, as well as daily activities such as walking to the store, taking the stairs or raking the leaves . . . Opportunities to accumulate physical activity during the school day include time spent in physical education class, classroom-based movement, recess, walking or biking to school, and recreational sport and play that occurs before, during, and after school.

(2010)

In other words, physical education exists as a distinct subject content area that is bound by state and local curricular standards as well as teacher certification requirements. On the other hand, physical activity could potentially mean just about any form of physical movement, thus opening the door for what might euphemistically be called 'creative accounting' when it comes to whether schools are meeting the physical activity requirements of the Wellness Policy legislation.

A number of states decided to use the Wellness Policy legislation to enact stronger physical education requirements. These states then had to decide what counts as adequate physical education. This became especially important for states like New York, California, Mississippi, Iowa, Nebraska and others that tie physical education credits to high school graduation. This situation lead to debates about, for example, whether recess time counted as physical education. Across the United States there currently exists a number of contradictory policies on this matter. In Texas, for example, the 2005 Senate Bill 42 states that it:

Encourages school districts to promote physical activity for children through classroom curricula for health and physical education. Allows the state board of education, by rule, to require students in kindergarten to grade nine to participate in up to 30 minutes of daily physical activity as part of a school district's physical education curriculum, through structured activity or during a school's daily recess.

(National Conference of State Legislators 2010)

In New York, however, recess may not count toward a student's physical education requirement. More specifically, the New York State Department of Education writes:

Recess may not be used to meet the physical education days/time requirement . . . The regulation is very specific on who may teach physical education: physical education must be taught by a certified physical education teacher or an elementary classroom teacher under the direction and supervision of a certified physical education teacher.

(2010)

The National Alliance for Nutrition and Activity has not clarified its position on whether recess qualifies as physical education, but they do outline what school personnel should be doing during recess to encourage physical activity among children: 'All elementary school students will have at least 20 minutes a day of supervised recess, preferably outdoors, during which schools should encourage moderate to vigorous physical activity verbally and through the provision of space and equipment' (2005: 16).

Statements about what should and should not count as physical education or official physical activity time in schools have proliferated. Our sense is that, like the previous quotes, they often serve to make the situation less clear rather than more clear. What, for example, does it mean to 'encourage moderate to vigorous physical activity'? Does this mean that teachers on playground duty must, on top of everything else, spend time looking for children who are not being sufficiently active? And what happened to the idea of recess as time for children to be by themselves and direct their own play?

The extent to which physical activity is necessary also seems dependent on the testing regime of the particular school. According to the National Alliance for Nutrition and Activity:

> Schools should discourage extended periods (i.e., periods of two or more hours) of inactivity. When activities, such as mandatory school-wide testing, make it necessary for students to remain indoors for long periods of time, schools should give students periodic breaks during which they are encouraged to stand and be moderately active.
>
> (2005: 16)

Apart from recess, another controversial issue has been whether participating in marching band should count towards a school's physical education and/or physical activity requirement. Consider the South Carolina Band Director's Association position statement on the issue:

> Education leaders are now confronted with emerging issues relating to physical fitness and life styles of today's youth, and the role played by the public education system in confronting these challenges. One such crisis is the nationwide obesity epidemic among adolescents, and the deterrence of this condition in developing productive citizens.
>
> (n.d.)

The South Carolina Band Director's Association go on to argue that:

> PE criteria requires a demonstration of competency in at least two movement forms. Band requires coordinated movement in multiple aspects of coordinated movement in all directions. To mention a few: forward march, backward march, slide movement, basic dance movement, horns up/down, marking time, precise group motion, instrument slides, flag coordination, step off

initiation, interval control, and more. The criteria attempts to develop active participants. Band not only develops active participants, it requires intense physical activity. The regime calls for calisthenics, stretching, running, and stationary exercises. The criteria require the development of an appropriate physical fitness program to achieve a desired level of personal fitness. Student band members not only design a program, they actually live it during their high school band experience. Marching band members engage in cardiovascular endurance, muscular strength and endurance, body composition in order to perform, and flexibility. Concert band members engage in a planned fitness exercise so as to meet the physical and respiratory challenges required of a performance. Assessment is monitored by the students and instructors.

(n.d.)

Other marching band advocates maintain that any student who wears a '40-pound tuba and walk[s] around at 120 beats a minute' (Drake 2002) will definitely be getting worthwhile exercise. However, not all educators feel similarly disposed. Opponents of the move often cite research like that of Strand and Sommer (2005), which shows a significant difference between the heart rates of individuals carrying heavy and light instruments. This study also showed that neither group (light or heavy) met the Surgeon General's recommendations for thirty minutes of daily moderate activity.

The California Association for Physical Education, Recreation and Dance have also weighed into the debates, taking a particularly strong view on the subject:

> Clearly recognizing the health, educational, and economical values of a citizenry that was equipped to engage in an active lifestyle, California's policy makers made sound decisions to include physical education in the required course of study for all students in grades 1–12 . . . Classes and activities that include some physical activity (marching band, JROTC, cheer, etc.) have important but distinctly different goals and objectives than physical education . . . However, these activities do not provide a comprehensive standards-based physical education experience and should not be allowed to fulfil the requirement for physical education.

(2009)

Avoiding the most important question

As trivial as debates about band practice and physical education might seem, school leaders must take them very seriously (see Ohio Department of Education 2010 for another example of official attempts to clarify these issues). Answers to what counts as physical activity and physical education all have significant curricular, personnel and budgetary implications. And yet the point to which we want to draw attention is that, of all the questions that school leaders must ask themselves in this legislative context, the one question that is not asked is whether any of the measures being debated will do anything to reduce obesity.

As the childhood obesity policy debate began to heat up in the United States, many interested organisations began to produce policy league tables. These tables were supposed to provide simple snapshots of which states had implemented the most rigorous obesity policies and which states were lagging behind. It soon became clear, however, that state legislatures were responding by passing legislation so that they could at least claim that they had a policy on, say, what foods could be sold in school cafeterias. Through all the debate about which were the leading and which were the failing states, we were able to find no discussion about the quality of these policies. In fact, there appears to have been no consideration of the accumulated research into school-based interventions whatsoever. In her book *Rethinking Thin*, Gina Kolata (2007) argues that research in this area has been conspicuously ignored, a point of view endorsed by the researchers she interviewed.

Why are these findings ignored? Our best answer is a mixture of anecdotal experience and speculation; there seems the world over to be a studied determination to believe that society's problems can simply be thrown at schools to be fixed. The naive hope that schools can work a kind of magic appears to die very hard and this is perhaps especially so if policy-makers are reluctant to take more direct measures. In other words, perhaps the fantasy of a school-based war on obesity persists precisely because policy-makers do not want to risk more controversial and politically unpopular courses of action. After all, the idea that schools can fix obesity appears to be a widely held, common-sense assumption that has spread even amongst the ranks of obesity researchers. In short, like all beliefs, no matter how farfetched, it persists only when people want it to be true.

For our part, we think that if existing research into schools and anti-obesity interventions counts for anything, there is little likelihood that existing policies will have any effect on American rates of childhood overweight and obesity. Nonetheless, we accept that some readers will not share our view and, instead, will argue that doing something is better than doing nothing. To these readers we would pose another series of questions: does the policy environment we have described in this chapter suggest a mature, concerted or co-ordinated approach to the problem of childhood obesity? What is the likelihood that American taxpayers are getting value for money from all this legislative activity? In short, how sound does the assumption that schools are a logical place to fight the war on obesity now appear?

Studying policy environments like that of the United States yields some contentious but, we think, plausible conclusions. Rather than being a sign that it has finally arrived as a pressing social policy priority, we would argue that assigning the obesity epidemic to schools is an indication of the contrary, that policy-makers do not believe childhood obesity is the 'drop everything' health crisis that some believe it to be. It is certainly difficult to imagine anyone who was determined to do something about, say, global warming, terrorism or the spread of infectious disease concluding that schools were the best or even a significant place to start. What schools do provide policy-makers is a cheap way of demonstrating that they have at least done something. With vague, unfunded policies in place, and with little or no accountability mechanism as follow-up, policy-makers can wash their hands of the problem and leave others to squabble over the details. And under the rhetorical cover of leaving local communities to develop 'local solutions', questions about policy efficacy can be completely avoided. We say again, if the problem were so serious and urgent, why would we leave it to committees of interested citizens and already busy teachers and their administrators?

The policy context that we have described presents a somewhat paradoxical picture. While the word 'crisis' is used liberally, and policies are being hastily developed and implemented to address the crisis, we hear the unmistakable sound of feet dragging. While the terms 'epidemic' and 'crisis' have created a wasteful sense of urgency in policy circles, it is a special kind of urgency, inclined to act without thinking, so that virtually all actions, no matter how varied or counter-intuitive, will do. Thus, the urgency for policy-makers is just as likely to be directed at meeting the demands for action rather than solving a problem that is seen as too difficult or just not a high enough priority. This should not surprise anyone. The histories of both party politics in general and school education in particular are littered with policy examples that were high on symbolic value but low on resources to oversee the planning, implementation and evaluation. It remains to be seen whether we have witnessed the high-water mark of school-based obesity policy in the United States or whether there is more to come. And yet we think there are already signs of resistance and that, weak as some current policies are, they may be more onerous and obtrusive than many people will tolerate.

6   Defenders of the truth

The 'empirical sceptics'

I chose the terms 'morality' and 'ideology' for the subtitle of *The Obesity Epidemic* with a precise goal in mind. What I was not trying to do was to show how obesity researchers, doctors, journalists and other commentators were cruel, stupid or dishonest. There are always exceptions, but then, as now, I did not believe the obesity epidemic was primarily a fabrication created by people with something to gain or an expression of one group's hostility or hatred of another group. My target was not people, but ways of thinking. As with this book, I was interested in the way pre-existing moral convictions and ideological commitments influence and shape what people believe, say and write. This is why my primary source of data has always been the words that researchers and other experts use. I look for moral and ideological traces in these words because this is one of the ways (although obviously not the only way) we might judge whether a given statement is credible. For example, it is clear to me that much of the hyperbole that surrounded children's use of televisions and computers grew from an underlying and long-standing cultural anxiety about technology and its effects on human minds and bodies. While new technologies bring with them the allure of a better, more comfortable future, they also generate nostalgia for an imagined past in which we lived more natural, robust and less alienated lives.

Closer to the concerns of this book, in previous chapters I have tried to show how certain ways of thinking about obesity fostered what, in the end, has become a world-wide movement, a kind of global group-think in which the terms 'crisis' and 'epidemic' have held sway. To reiterate, this does not mean that I think people talked about children dying younger than their parents or about obesity increasing at accelerating rates (when, in fact, rates appear to have slowed) because they were dishonest or stupid. My argument is that they said these things, by and large, because they allowed themselves to think about obesity in received ways and because 'crises' and 'epidemics' have become the default register in which industrialised societies have learnt to talk about many of the challenges they face. In fact, it is absolutely clear that some obesity experts have used the language of crisis in order to attract attention to their cause. This fact by itself does not make them dishonest or maliciously opportunistic. It simply underlines the unremarkable point that people who talk and write about obesity, no matter what opinions they express, are shaped by the culture in which they live.

In this chapter and Chapter 7 I make what to some readers will seem a strange, even perverse change of direction. Having made a case for the obesity epidemic's statistical and political end in Chapters 2, 3, 4 and 5, I now want to discuss an ending of a different kind. In its early years the obesity epidemic travelled a mostly uncontested passage from the pages of academic journals to the nightly television news. Its overheated rhetoric notwithstanding, it was presented as a common-sense story with which few could or did disagree. For a few years at least, it enjoyed a gloss of consensus. This period of uncontested dominance is now over.

The emergence of writers and commentators whom I will collectively call the 'obesity sceptics' cover a surprisingly wide moral and ideological spectrum and it is partly this diversity that makes them interesting. Taken together, they ask us to consider the obesity epidemic in particular ways by offering us explanations of its emergence – Why did it happen? – and suggesting different kinds of responses to it. I now want to take the reader on a kind of guided tour in which I provide an account of the arguments different obesity sceptics make. So, although what follows will not please all readers, my purpose here is, in part, merely descriptive.

I use the term 'obesity sceptics' partly for convenience to talk about a disparate set of writers. In their different ways they have sought to argue against part or all of the dominant obesity story: that obesity rates have gone up alarmingly in recent decades, that this increase represents an international health crisis and that radical and far-reaching actions need to be taken to ameliorate the looming disaster. While it is true that a small number of academic dissidents had written on the subject in the latter part of the twentieth century, my focus in this chapter is on those who have come to prominence in the wake of the obesity epidemic post-2000 and, for the most part, have not written primarily for scientific and medical journals. These are the people who have attempted to bring obesity scepticism to a wider audience. And although I do not claim to provide a comprehensive account, I do attempt to summarise what I see as the dominant schools of thought in obesity scepticism.

The voices of obesity scepticism have multiplied in recent years, producing a vibrant and much-needed counter to the dominant story. But it is also true that sceptics, no less than alarmists, often think in ways that are the product and prisoner of pre-existing biases. What follows is an attempt to subject the thinking of sceptics to the same kind of scrutiny we should apply to all areas of knowledge. While, at least to me, this would seem a reasonable and important undertaking, the arguments of sceptics have not yet been seriously tested for at least two reasons. First, mainstream obesity science and medicine dwarf the ranks of the sceptics and have mostly been able to ignore the arguments of sceptics. Second, to the extent that there has been any debate between the two sides, sceptics have tended to present themselves as a unified David in opposition to the mainstream's Goliath. Beyond uncritically referring to each other's work, there has been virtually no internal dialogue between sceptics because to do so would threaten solidarity in their battles with obesity alarmism.

Solidarity, though, is a poor substitute for healthy self-examination and the remainder of this book is an initial attempt to foster a spirit of robust dialogue amongst sceptics. More than this, though, while I have my own opinions about the obesity epidemic, I am not primarily interested in converting readers to my point of view. Rather, I am attempting to contribute to debate and understanding so that, to borrow a phrase popular amongst philosophers, we might 'think well' about the issue. A more enlightened approach to obesity is impossible without rigorous and robust argument-making and, at times, a critical engagement with each other's ideas.

About truth

One final point of clarification is necessary before embarking on this survey of obesity scepticism. I start from a position of agnosticism towards the truth about obesity. In previous work I have been careful to avoid definitive pronouncements about what is really going on with the body weights and health of Western populations. To begin with, obesity research, much of it epidemiological and based on self-report data, is a notoriously inexact business. For example, there is still no consensus about even such fundamental issues as whether average Western per-person caloric consumption has gone up, gone down or stayed the same in recent decades. I have also learnt that what might look like common-sense assumptions are constantly being called into question by research. For instance, it is widely acknowledged that conclusive empirical evidence is lacking to support the idea that obese children and adults generally consume more calories than thinner children and adults.

What I take to be the inherent uncertainty of obesity research goes right through to the most important questions of all, such as what level of health risk attaches to BMI scores above the so-called 'normal' cut-off point of 25. My position is that the real risks of being classified as overweight or obese have, on balance, probably been exaggerated. But I also accept that the question of health risk is not easily resolved and that the results of research tend to be open to a wide range of interpretations. What seems most important, then, is not so much to prove who is right, but why, given radical uncertainty, different people choose to believe what they appear to believe. For example, how is it possible that large sections of the obesity science communities could make literally thousands of confidently apocalyptic predictions about the future of the obesity epidemic without the support of a secure knowledge base? But we might also ask what motivates an obesity sceptic to announce categorically that body weight has virtually no bearing on health whatsoever. Both positions seem unwise to me.

So, at the risk of frustrating readers looking for reliable truths, one of my core analytical techniques is to look for assertions of certainty where I think they are unjustified. In fact, taken together, if this book and its predecessor make any one single claim, it is that the business of trying to understand obesity research calls for a kind of alchemy, where the mercury of uncertainty must magically be transformed into the gold of truth. The argument that I now want to prosecute is that this is as true of obesity sceptics as it has been of the alarmists.

Letting science speak

Collectively, I call the sceptics I discuss in this chapter 'empirical sceptics'. This is certainly not because I see them as especially empirical or scientific in their methods. In a few cases in particular, this is very far from the case. In part, the term is intended ironically, although I would want to avoid tipping into sarcasm. The salient point is that these sceptics claim to base their arguments on 'what the data says' and they see themselves as more objective and truthful than those they criticise. It is their ostentatious self-styling as guardians of scientific truth which is important to me here. While Chapter 7 deals with writers who tend to see the obesity epidemic as the product of 'normal' science, those in this chapter see it as a scientific perversion.

Perhaps the best-known books written by obesity sceptics are Glen Gaesser's (2002) *Big Fat Lies: The Truth About Your Weight and Your Health*, Paul Campos's (2004a) *The Obesity Myth: Why America's Obsession with Weight is Hazardous to your Health* and J. Eric Oliver's (2006) *Fat Politics: The Real Story Behind America's Obesity Epidemic* (see also Campos, Saguy, Ernsberger, Oliver and Gaesser 2006 for an example of these three authors writing together). Together, these works have helped to establish obesity scepticism as a legitimate intellectual position and popularise sceptical arguments. Most crucial of all, they have each contributed to building the case against seeing obesity per se as a disease, demonstrating that the health risks of fatness are, at the very least, highly debatable. In many respects, Gaesser was the groundbreaker, presenting his ideas both in scholarly journals and on daytime American television. More recently, Campos has been a tireless, acerbic and superbly articulate warrior for the sceptical position in his extensive print an electronic media work. All three writers have been indispensable sources of data and analysis in developing my own work.

Right from the front covers of Gaesser, Campos and Oliver's books it is difficult to miss their explicit use of polar opposites: 'truth' versus 'myth', 'facts' versus 'lies' and 'the real story' versus 'politics'. The cover of my copy of Gaesser's book beckons readers to 'Learn the astonishing facts'. The message is clear. While Jan Wright and I argued in *The Obesity Epidemic* that morality and ideology filled in the very large gaps created by a radically inconclusive scientific literature, for Gaesser, Campos and Oliver there appear to be no gaps; objective scientific truth is there for any honest person who cares to look at the evidence.

For example, around the time of the release of *The Obesity Myth*, Campos published a series of articles in newspapers around the world under headlines like 'Big fat lie' and 'The big fat con story'.[1] In one of these articles he writes:

> What I have found may prove hard for some to swallow: save for exceptions involving truly extreme cases, the medical literature simply does not support

---

1 I fully appreciate the possibility that some or all of these titles may not have been Campos's choice. In 2005 I wrote a newspaper article for The Age newspaper in Australia. The title of my article was changed, without my know knowledge, to 'The obesity myth'.

the claim that higher than average weight is a significant independent health risk. What it actually demonstrates is, first, that the association between increased weight and increased health risk is weak, and disappears altogether when confounding variables are taken into account; and second, that public health programmes which attempt to make "overweight" and "obese" people thinner are, for a variety of reasons, likely to do more harm than good. In short, the current war on fat is an irrational outburst of cultural hysteria, unsupported by sound science.

(Campos 2004b: 20)

Are obesity scientists 'liars' involved in a 'con'? Is it fair to describe them as 'irrational' or in the grip of 'cultural hysteria'? Do we really know that most obesity-related public health interventions will do more harm than good? Notice also Campos's assertion that 'sound science' is on his side and the implication that he will speak on its behalf. In *The Obesity Myth* itself Campos goes even further:

This book documents how the current barrage of claims about the supposedly devastating medical and economic consequences of "excess" weight is a product of greed, junk science, and outright bigotry . . . The war on fat is unique in American history in that it represents the first concerted attempt to transform the vast majority of the nation's citizens into social pariahs, to be pitied and scorned until weapons of mass destruction can be found that will rid them of their shameful condition.

(2004b: xvii)

In many similar passages throughout *The Obesity Myth* Campos rejects the idea that the stigmatisation of overweight and obese people might be an unintended consequence of the war on fatness rather than its explicit purpose. And in case readers were in any doubt about what he sees as their motives, Campos dismisses the possibility that health authorities might have the health of overweight and obese people uppermost in their minds:

The health establishment's constant barrage of scientifically baseless propaganda regarding the relationship between weight and health constitutes nothing less than egregious abuse of public trust. This propaganda has played a key role in creating a culture that makes tens of millions of people miserable about their bodies: Worse yet, it has done so for crass economic motives. The war on fat, which is supposedly about making all of us healthy, is really about making some of us rich.

(2004b: xix)

His position could scarcely be more clear: what we have here is not a difference of scientific opinion but a deceit, a fraud or, as Campos puts it, an 'abuse of trust'.

From here on, Campos continually describes the 'propaganda' of the 'medical and health establishments' as 'lies' and his own pronouncements as 'facts'.

Campos writes, 'Many of the *facts* in this section are likely to astonish anyone who has relied on the mass media for information on this issue' (2004b: xxi, my emphasis) and later, 'I am an advocate for truth, and its indispensable partner, honesty' (2004b: 5).

Like Campos, Oliver and Gaesser blame something called the 'health establishment' for the obesity epidemic, although Oliver at least makes some effort to be more specific about who the 'health establishment' is: 'Over the past two decades, a handful of scientists, doctors, and health officials have actively campaigned to define our growing weight as an obesity epidemic' (Oliver 2006: 5). Although not spelt out, if anything, Gaesser's 'health establishment' and 'medical establishment' (he refers to both without clarification) seem to encompass a somewhat broader sweep of the medical and research communities than those of either Campos or Oliver. Gaesser also takes a particular swipe at the fashion and fitness industries for going out their way to construct body fat as both aesthetically undesirable and a sign of moral failing.

Oliver differs slightly from Campos in that he is prepared to concede that some proponents of the obesity epidemic have acted with 'good intentions' and 'sincerely believe that having too much fat leads to harm and disease, even if the scientific evidence is inconclusive' (Oliver 2006: 6). However, Oliver then goes on to make it clear that the health establishment's pecuniary self-interest and hatred of fat people, particularly if they are poor or non-white, are at the heart of the matter: 'For many people, trumpeting the "problem of obesity" is an opportunity for them to express both their own moral superiority and their latent class snobbery and racism' (2006: 7).

It is worth pausing for a moment to consider what is meant by the 'health establishment', a term all three authors use regularly. This is obviously a rather loaded term, but there is more to this than meets the eye. We need to keep in mind that because Campos and Oliver in particular want to us to see the obesity epidemic as the work of a group of corrupt and misguided individuals, their argument needs a villain. In their formulation, what we have is a scandal in need of a mastermind, a crime in need of a criminal. Enter the 'health establishment'.

Gaesser, Campos and Oliver's argument would be much more difficult to make if the obesity epidemic were – as I think it is (see Chapter 8 for discussion on this point) – a broad scientific and social movement, encompassing a significant portion of a large and diverse research community. After all, if many people are involved then the idea of a calculated conspiracy begins to look much less plausible. It is particularly revealing that beyond statements like those quoted above, Gaesser, Campos and Oliver never really identify who they mean by the 'health establishment'. Of course, being any more specific would invite the challenge of having to name names and actually prove the charge of corrupt behaviour. On the other hand, casting the net too wide raises the problem of undermining the picture of a kind of health mafia working maliciously behind the scenes. In short, the idea of a 'health establishment' is both sufficiently vague not to draw too much attention to itself and narrow enough to be a suitable villain in Gaesser, Campos and Oliver's morality play. It is surely also not a coincidence that, of the three, Gaesser's 'health establishment' appears to be the largest and that the idea of a self-interested conspiracy is much less prominent in his analysis.

It appears to be Gaesser, Campos and Oliver's determination to be seen as obesity's truth tellers that motivates the construction of their 'health establishment' straw man. If the truth of obesity is as self-evident as they say it is, and the lies of the 'health establishment' so egregious, then the only possible explanation is a conspiracy. After all, if the truth about obesity were, instead, murky, complex and contested then Campos's claim that the obesity epidemic is 'a product of greed, junk science, and outright bigotry' might, itself, begin to sound more than a little hysterical.

Despite their attacks on the honesty and competency of obesity researchers, Gaesser, Campos and Oliver manage to find a single needle in the haystack of obesity research in the shape of the epidemiologist Steven Blair, a name we will encounter a number of times in this chapter. Blair is best known for studying the effects of exercise on people's body weight and health. Readers may recall (see Chapter 2) his prediction that American physical inactivity, as opposed to obesity, is 'the biggest public health problem of the 21st century'.

It is difficult to be precise or prescriptive about the health benefits of physical activity and over the years many researchers have been prepared to dismiss the claims of exercise advocates as mere self-righteous fanaticism. There are many reasons for this controversy, but the most obvious reason is that it is extremely difficult to control for all the variables that may contribute to a person's long-term health outcomes and, thereby, isolate and measure the effect of physical activity. For example, more physically active people tend to be wealthier and live in areas that confer a wide range of potential health benefits. Physically active people are also more likely to exhibit a range of other behaviours thought to be health enhancing. In addition, the medium- and long-term health benefits of physical activity are often extrapolated from large self-report studies, where the amount of physical activity that people do has not even been directly measured.

The very fact that the case in favour of physical activity tends to rely so heavily on imprecise data, which are derived from samples numbering in the thousands and sometimes tens of thousands, leads to a number of uncomfortable conclusions. For example, against the assertion that it is a universally and unproblematically health-enhancing behaviour, one possibility is that physical activity has very different health effects on different people. It may also be that, rather than protecting against ill-health generally, physical activity has a different effect on different forms of ill-health, an effect which may, in turn, vary from person to person. It is also very hard to know how much physical activity people actually do and direct empirical evidence that rising obesity has been caused by decreasing activity levels is scarce. Uncertainty about population (or, indeed, individual) physical activity levels turns all but the most generalised statement about the health benefits of physical activity into mere speculation; if you do not know how much physical activity people are doing, how can you be sure how beneficial it is?

Nonetheless, Gaesser, Campos and Oliver all rely heavily on Blair's research that appears to show that a person's fitness and physical activity levels are more important than their body weight. This leads to the by now quite well-known assertion that fat and fit is actually healthier than thin and unfit. All three authors assert that while physical activity has a large bearing on a person's health, body weight is close to meaningless except at the extremes.

The problem here is that these ideas have been regularly disputed on scientific grounds. There is a straightforward reply from the obesity alarmist camp that says that Blair's research does not implicate fatness because the BMI is simply not sensitive enough to account for actual adiposity and particularly the effect of 'bad fat', which is found on the chest and abdomen (Romero-Corral et al. 2006). In addition, it is impossible to say whether it is a person's fitness level or the physical activity they did to get fit that confers health benefit. In any case, a widely cited meta-analysis (Katzmarzyk, Janssen and Arden 2003) of studies published between 1965 and 2003 concluded that body weight and physical activity are independent mortality risk factors, a point emphasised since by other researchers (for example Berentzen and Sørensen 2007). I want to be clear here that I am not endorsing Blair's position or that of his critics, but rather drawing attention to the way Gaesser, Campos and Oliver create the impression of certainty about this area of research when no such certainty exists.

It is also worth pointing that, whatever we might think about the quality of their work, a number of well-known researchers have recently announced their conclusion that the obesity epidemic has largely been the result of increased caloric intake rather than decreasing levels of physical activity (Bleich, Cutler, Murray and Adams 2008; EurekAlert 2009). I have to say that I remain non-plussed that anyone still thinks a relatively simple answer to the diet-or-exercise question is possible and I remain utterly agnostic on the matter. Nonetheless, Gaesser, Campos and Oliver all either imply or state categorically that the obesity epidemic is more the result of decreasing physical activity than dietary intake.

What is more puzzling though is that, despite Gaesser, Campos and Oliver's claim that we are in the middle of a corrupt and hysterical panic over body weight, they all appear to align themselves with Blair's dire predictions about physical activity. All three warn that we are doing insufficient exercise and not eating the right foods. In effect, they seem simply to have swapped one epidemic (obesity) for a couple of others: inactivity and poor diets. Both Campos and Gaesser want public policy to be directed towards increasing physical activity and improving people's diets rather than focusing on weight loss per se. Gaesser repeatedly argues that it is fat in the diet not on the body about which we should be worried and that Americans are eating much more fat than they used to, itself an assertion which is regularly contradicted in the research literature (for example Bray and Popkin 1998; Gregg et al. 2005; Hill and Peters 1998; Kennedy, Bowman and Powell 1999).

Oliver's formulation is only subtlely different. He concurs that people are doing less physical activity, but wants to draw attention to a particular aspect of the American diet:

Americans are not consuming more calories because of how much they are eating during their meals. (Americans consume only slightly more calories in their meals today than they did in the 1970s.) Rather, Americans are consuming more calories because of how much they are eating *in between* their meals. The real culprit behind our increasing weight is snacking.

(2006: 9, emphasis in original)

At this point some might argue that the distinction Gaesser, Campos and Oliver want to draw between body weight on the one hand and exercise and diet on the other hand is an important one. But is it? On a practical level one of the most obvious real-world effects of the obesity epidemic has been a proliferation of public health campaigns imploring us to exercise more and eat healthier food. In schools all over the Western world the obesity epidemic has been the catalyst for programs designed to make children change their diets, exercise more and, in some cases, increase their fitness in order to avoid some form of sanction. For all Gaesser, Campos and Oliver's claims to be heretics and the enemies of the 'health establishment', how different are they? In the following passage from *The Obesity Myth* Campos says that 'the prosecutors in the case against fat' have 'indicted the wrong parties':

Americans are too sedentary. We do eat too much junk that isn't good for us, because it's quick and cheap and easier than the alternative of spending time and money to prepare food that is both good for us and satisfies our cravings. A rational public health policy would focus on those issues, not on weight, which isn't the problem, any more than diet and diet drugs would be the solution, even if they actually made people thin.

(2004a: 248)

My reaction to this is that the 'rational public health policy' that Campos wants, focusing on nutrition and physical activity, is not some distant Utopia; it is the public health policy environment that we currently have.

But there is an even deeper problem with Gaesser, Campos and Oliver's case against the obesity epidemic and the 'health establishment'. While it is true that there are many obesity experts who spend a great deal of their time emphasising the risks of excess body weight per se, what Gaesser, Campos and Oliver seem to overlook is that, by and large, these people also spend a lot of their time advocating for more physical activity and better diets. In other words, the people calling for a war on fat – which Gaesser, Campos and Oliver do not want – are largely the same people calling for policies to increase physical activity and better nutrition – which Gaesser, Campos and Oliver do want. Although literally hundreds of examples could be offered, Chakravarthy and Booth (2003), in the journal *Archives of Pediatrics and Adolescent Medicine*, illustrate this point perfectly. The article, 'Inactivity and inaction: we can't afford either', is replete with the kind of obesity rhetoric that Gaesser, Campos and Oliver could surely have no truck with:

Overwhelming data show that an obese child has a high probability of becoming an obese adult. Of children who eventually become either overweight or obese as adults, approximately one third do so before age 20 years; the remaining two thirds become overweight or obese after age 20 years. Pediatric obesity-related hospital costs have increased 3-fold during the last 20 years, reaching $127 million per year.

(Chakravarthy and Booth 2003: 731)

And yet, like the vast majority of obesity researchers, Chakravarthy and Booth see no distinction between what they see as the twin epidemics of obesity and inactivity:

Given that children were less sedentary 50 years ago, we believe that by instituting similar lifestyle modifications (watching less TV, eating fewer higher-calorie fast foods, and being more physically active), the current rising physical inactivity and obesity epidemics can be thwarted.

(2003: 731)

And later:

Considering the public health ramifications of obesity and physical inactivity, primary prevention of these epidemics is not a choice; it is mandatory. The cost of inaction from a humanitarian, clinical, socio-economic, and health care dollar perspective is a price that we cannot afford.

(2003: 732)

In effect, what Gaesser, Campos and Oliver ask us to believe is that when it comes to body weight, mainstream obesity medicine and science are corrupt, dishonest, incompetent and bigoted, while, at the same time, they are able to appreciate the importance of physical activity and diet with perfect clarity. And while Gaesser, Campos and Oliver are apparently convinced that the idea of the obesity epidemic has largely been fuelled by the dirty money of the pharmaceutical and weight loss industries, the idea of an 'epidemic of inactivity', *à la* Steven Blair, is simply an untainted and irrefutable scientific fact. Gaesser, Campos and Oliver seem unaware that some obesity scientists actually concede the point that more physical activity and better diets may have comparable health benefits to weight loss. More important though, in trying to turn the obesity epidemic into an outrageous conspiracy, they exaggerate the difference between themselves and the people they criticise. This, in turn, constructs the truth about the health risks of excess body weight as a battle between the forces of good and evil when it may, instead, simply be a run-of-the-mill difference of opinion and scientific interpretation, a much less dramatic and commercially exploitable state of affairs.

Why do they do this? In the next section we will see how the idea of an epidemic of inactivity is used for straightforward ideological reasons. However, for Gaesser, Campos and Oliver the answer is less clear. My sense of it is that, in the context of their obvious strategy to paint themselves as the tellers of unbiased scientific truth, Gaesser, Campos and Oliver found themselves needing to replace one set of scientific claims with another. In other words, it is probably more difficult to claim the scientific high ground while also offering only an equivocal 'I don't know' as your scientific counter-argument. Paraphrasing the famous knife scene in Paul Hogan's movie *Crocodile Dundee*, they decided to tell their audiences: 'That's not the truth. *This* is the truth!'

Obesity and the market

I now turn to a second group of obesity sceptics, whose arguments, in subtle and fascinating ways, both echo and contradict Gaesser, Campos and Oliver. Much has been written about this group, which is made up of a loose coalition of free-market libertarians and food industry lobby groups. This is particularly true of the lobbyists, who are well known for attempting to defend the practices of the major food corporations (for discussions of the activity of the lobbyists, see Brownell and Horgen 2004; Brownell and Warner 2009; Bunting 2002; Nestle 2000, 2002a, 2002b). Oliver's (2006) *Fat Politics* provides a particularly compelling account of their activities, from the funding of research journals and professional organizations to their tireless lobbying of politicians against industry regulation.

Although writers like Gaesser, Campos and Oliver and food industry lobbyists have overlapping concerns – they are both intent on arguing that far too much has been made of rising obesity levels – Gaesser, Campos and Oliver are keen to distance themselves from industry groups. This is hardly surprising; they want to present themselves as the honest face of scientific truth rather than the stooges of corporate power. However, rather than dismissing them out of hand, there is value in listening to the kinds of arguments the industry lobbyists and their libertarian cousins make. This is not to say that their arguments are more credible than other obesity sceptics. In fact, many of their claims are extremely dubious. What is instructive, though, is the way free-market scepticism both overlaps and differs from the work of those discussed in the previous section. In other words, by mapping the contrasting truth claims of different sceptics we are better able to detect the ideological and moral forces at work.

To begin, let us consider *An Epidemic of Obesity Myths* (hereafter *AEOM*) (Center for Consumer Freedom 2005), a publication of the Washington D. C.-based and food industry-funded Center for Consumer Freedom.[2] *AEOM* devotes much of its attention to critiquing some of the more hyperbolic claims made by obesity science and the mass media. In particular, it spends many pages discussing the Centers for Disease Control and Prevention controversy concerning the number of American deaths attributable to excess body weight (see Chapter 2). Although complete with photographs and light-hearted cartoons, *AEOM*'s pages actually make reference to a lengthy list of academic publications, all of which are footnoted, and they dedicate a significant amount of space to discussing research-related issues. Although clearly intended for a wide audience, the writer(s) of *AEOM* have gone to considerable trouble to at least give the impression of scientific rigour.

In many ways there is little to distinguish the approach and overall arguments put forward by *AEOM* and Gaesser, Campos and Oliver. Each attempts to refute the science of the obesity epidemic by providing their own summaries of the

2 This publication has been published and updated a number of times. I refer here to the 2005 iteration.

scientific evidence. Each attempts to present the obesity epidemic as a conspiracy perpetrated by a self-interested group of health workers, researchers and officials. Like Gaesser, Campos and Oliver, *AEOM* also leaps enthusiastically on the work of Steven Blair and announces that it is lack of exercise, not body fat, that is the enemy. The contradiction created by embracing Blair's work and the idea that sedentary behaviour is the epidemic that obesity is not, however, is even starker in *AEOM*. Having spent the first seventy or so pages lampooning and dismissing the idea that obesity kills 400,000 Americans every year, *AEOM*'s hitherto hyper-sceptical approach to epidemiological research suddenly evaporates:

> Physical inactivity causes a tremendous burden of disease and death. Researchers commissioned by the President's Council on Physical Fitness and Sports coined the phrase "Sedentary Death Syndrome." And no wonder. In 2000, *The Journal of Applied Physiology* reported that approximately "250,000 deaths per year in the United States are premature due to physical inactivity." The Active Living by Design program indicates that "34% of coronary heart disease deaths can be attributed to physical inactivity; physically inactive adults are nearly twice as likely than those who are active to have coronary heart disease." A study in the journal *Medicine and Science in Sports and Exercise* reports: "Sedentary living is responsible for about one-third of deaths due to coronary heart disease, colon cancer, and diabetes." And according to an article in *The New England Journal of Medicine*, the risk of death among the least fit is four times greater than it is among the most fit.
> (Centre for Consumer Freedom 2005: 82–83)

The complexities that are glossed over in statements like this are myriad. It is simply impossible to know with any degree of certainty how much death and disease is caused by people's physical inactivity, a point that is widely acknowledged in the research literature. Even more obvious, perhaps, is that physically active people tend to differ from less active people on many social indicators, such as income and educational attainment. These differences make it extremely difficult to determine whether health outcomes are caused by the physical activity that people do or some other factor.

As I will stress a number of times in this chapter, though, it is theoretically possible that assertions like those made in relation to physical activity in *AEOM* may turn out to be incontrovertible scientific truths. I think this is doubtful, but this possibility must be allowed. However, more pertinent to my focus on the rhetorical techniques used by obesity sceptics is *how* this case is made. For example, *AEOM* reproduces a number of quotes from academic journals – a large number of which are by the same author, Steven Blair – that appear to claim that since average caloric consumption has not gone up in the United States, the cause of rising obesity must be declining physical activity. With these quotes lined up, one after the other over a few pages, the impression of evidence stacking up higher and higher is created. But there is an obvious point to make: just as many quotes claiming the opposite – that because there has been no change in physical activity levels, the obesity epidemic must be the result of changing diets – can easily be found in the scientific literature (for examples and discussion of the schizophrenic nature of the research on this issue see Gard and Wright 2005: Chapter 6). By quoting selectively from the literature, the authors of *AEOM* appear to want readers to believe that science speaks with one voice on the relative contribution of food and physical activity to rising rates of obesity. This is plainly misleading.

The same applies to its treatment of the contribution of food environments to obesity. *AEOM* offers a handful of quotes that appear to exonerate the marketing of food to children as well as the obvious and widespread changes to the general food environments of Western countries. In a brief section that bears the intentionally ironic title 'Toxic Food Environment', evidence from only one scientific paper is offered:

> The so-called 'toxic food environment' is often blamed for contributing to American obesity. Activists and academics claim that the number of convenient, inexpensive food options makes it too easy to eat. But leading research published in *The International Journal of Obesity* in 2005 determined that 'there was no relationship between availability of eating places and prevalence of obesity.'
>
> (Center for Consumer Freedom 2005: 100)

As with most research into the causes of the obesity epidemic, research on food marketing and food environments is consistently inconsistent and equivocal. However, this does not mean, as *AEOM* suggests, that there is no debate to be had and that there is no case against modern food cultures. For example, many researchers point out that there can be no doubt that more and more high-calorie food and drink *has* been produced in recent decades. These extra calories, they essentially argue, must be going somewhere (Caballero 2007; French, Story and Jeffery 2001). There are also well-known problems with the extent to which people, especially children, reliably report to researchers the food and drink they have actually consumed. Once again though, a difficult and complex debate is sidestepped by *AEOM*, apparently in order to create the impression of scientific unanimity.

AEOM does the same when it claims that Americans consume no more calories than they used to. As we have seen, this is in direct contrast to Gaesser, Campos and Oliver, who all say the opposite. So, while Oliver attempts to implicate between meal snacking for rising obesity, *AEOM* wants its readers to accept that changes to the way food is advertised, sold and consumed have had no impact whatsoever on population body weights or health. The answers, it argues, can only be found on the physical activity side of the equation.

But like Gaesser, Campos and Oliver, *AEOM* blames the obesity epidemic on a relatively small group of corrupt and compromised individuals and organisations. By way of evidence, it lists the pharmaceutical and weight-loss industry sponsors of some of the most well-known obesity researchers and accuses these people of sliding 'from science to activism' (Center for Consumer Freedom 2005: 72). In light of this accusation, it would be interesting to hear how the authors of *AEOM* would describe their own work if not as activism. This question is not addressed and readers are simply expected to accept that pharmaceutical and weight-loss industry sponsorship is utterly corrupting while their own sponsorship from 'restaurants, food companies, and consumers' seeks no more than to 'promote personal responsibility and protect consumer choice' (Center for Consumer Freedom 2005: 1).

Written by Patrick Basham, Gio Gori and John Luik (2006), *Diet Nation: Exposing the Obesity Crusade* takes us the short distance from *AEOM*'s industry spin to all-out ideological warfare. *Diet Nation* is one of the most detailed and thorough critiques of obesity science that I have encountered. It is also amongst the most politically committed.

I have listened to radio interviews with Patrick Basham and it is clear that he, like Gaesser, Campos and Oliver, wants to distance himself from the industry lobbyists. In fact, this is sufficiently important to the authors of *Diet Nation* for them to use its acknowledgements page to tell readers who they were *not* supported by: 'The food and beverage industry has had neither input into nor influence upon the planning, research, writing or editing stages of this project' (Basham, Gori and Luik 2006: 7). Is this a case of protesting too much? *Diet Nation* certainly comes to much the same conclusions as *AEOM* and the two documents identify many of the same villains in the ubiquitous 'health establishment', who are 'driven by enormous amounts of self-interest' (Basham, Gori and Luik 2006: 43–44). In fact, after reading *Diet Nation* one is tempted to conclude that the authors' protestations about having no connections with industry are there precisely because they make the same arguments as the industries by which they have supposedly not been influenced.

For example, the authors of *Diet Nation* go to extraordinary lengths to argue that, whatever else we might say about the obesity epidemic, we cannot blame food or the companies that make and advertise it. The book returns again and again to the standard industry argument, used for decades by tobacco companies, that advertising only ever affects people's choice of brands, not the kinds of products they desire. This will be news to anyone familiar with the history of advertising during the twentieth century and the way fast food and soft drink companies openly and explicitly sought to use advertising to create new demand for their previously non-existent products (for some historical perspective on this issue see McQueen 2001; for a more recent analysis see Simon 2006). Basham and colleagues also have absolutely no sympathy for any parent who feels that food advertising makes it more difficult to control children's diets. After all, if advertising does not stimulate demand for new products, as the authors claim, it is difficult to know how advertising for, say, fast food restaurants could ever have any effect on children. Nonetheless, *Diet Nation* makes the paradoxical demand that parents need to educate children to resist advertising that, the book claims, has no impact on the types of food children prefer in the first place.

If there is a difference between the industry-sponsored scepticism of *AEOM* and that of *Diet Nation*, it is not so much in substance, but in style. For *AEOM* there is no ideological battle to be won. It presents itself as concerned only with people's freedom to buy whatever food products when and where they want and claims that a small group of obesity experts have simply been paid to lie about the causes and health risks of obesity. In other words, there is a 'motherhood' quality to its case, a studied reasonableness designed to strike a reassuring tone and avoid too many hard rhetorical edges that might alienate some readers. After all, who could not be for consumer choice and against the corruption of science?

The delicacy of these rhetorical maneuverings is completely absent from *Diet Nation*. Although at one point it claims that the obesity epidemic is 'the work of a small number of people' (Basham, Gori and Luik 2006: 42), this is a rare show of self-restraint. For the authors, the obesity epidemic is nothing less than a fully-blown attack by what they call 'obesity crusaders' on individual liberty, democracy and capitalism itself. This, of course, stretches plausibility; if the obesity crusade really were the work of a 'small number of people', it is difficult to see how it could, at the same time, amount to a serious threat to the foundations of Western civilisation. And while the word 'socialism' is hardly used, the reader is left in little doubt that this is what Basham, Gori and Luik believe drives the enemy. Early in the book the authors assert that we must resist the claims of obesity crusaders because of '. . . the significant risk that many of the policy proposals to prevent obesity will erode further individual liberty by enhancing the State's exclusive power to define what constitutes a good life' (Basham, Gori and Luik 2006: 14). Later, the problem with the war on obesity is described as '. . . its enormous potential for eroding individual liberty through employing the engine of the State, particularly its propaganda and regulatory powers, once again to define and enforce a single vision of what constitutes a good life' (Basham, Gori and Luik 2006: 22–23). Towards the end of the book the obesity crusaders are '. . . heads-buried-in-the-empirical-sand, Leninist-minded academics, policymakers and regulators' (Basham, Gori and Luik 2006: 220).

That *Diet Nation*'s enemies should be 'Leninist-minded academics' is less surprising if one bothers to find out who its authors are. Patrick Basham is a founding director of the conservative Democracy Institute and is connected to free-market and right-wing think tanks like the Cato Institute. John Luik has connections with similar organisations, such as the Fraser Institute and the Niagara Institute, and has for many years written and campaigned on behalf of the tobacco industry.

If nothing else, *Diet Nation* is an example of how one's own ideological zeal can breed overheated imaginings of equally zealous opponents. Over the following pages I will attempt to justify this claim but, in a nutshell, when Basham, Gori and Luik talk about the 'obesity crusaders', they describe an incurably stupid and insatiably evil enemy. It is an enemy that is impossible to square with the world of obesity research and advocacy that I have engaged with and criticised over the last ten years.

I have already described *Diet Nation*'s attempts to exonerate food advertising. This is contentious enough and the authors completely avoid any discussion of the large body of writing about the sophisticated tactics used by food advertisers to influence children's behaviours, desires and tastes. It is not that these tactics are defended; they are simply not mentioned. However, the obesity crusaders are not only guilty of misunderstanding and exaggerating the effect of food advertising on children. According to *Diet Nation*, if it is not obvious now, 'It will soon become crystal clear that the war on fat is inherently a war on the food and beverage industry' (Basham, Gori and Luik 2006: 233). This startling claim rests on the assertion that the obesity research community constantly plays down the role of physical activity and sedentary living while grossly exaggerating the role of food:

> At the core of the obesity crusaders' story is an account of why there is suddenly so much obesity everywhere in the world. The answer to this question is that obesity is largely, though not completely, the result of a contrived food environment, an environment of unhealthy, inexpensive and heavily promoted foods served in enormous proportions; an environment engineered by the food industry. The problem is not one of caloric expenditure, which might just as well explain obesity, but one of consumption.
>
> (Basham, Gori and Luik 2006: 129)

It is true enough that these are some of the things one finds written in journal articles. It is also true that a small number of obesity scientists favour increased food consumption over declining physical activity levels as an explanation for the obesity epidemic. But there are also those who agree precisely with Basham, Gori and Luik's position that physical activity, not food, explains the obesity epidemic (for example Anderssen et al. 2008). In fact, the relative contribution of food and physical inactivity is a matter of spirited debate in the research literature, while the vast majority of commentators simply assume that both factors have played a role. In a standard rendering of the problem, Julie L. Gerberding, then director of the CDC and leading obesity 'crusader', testified to a United States Senate Committee in 2008 that 'No single cause or factor is to blame for the epidemic of obesity among children and adolescents. Indeed, many factors have contributed to the unfavorable trends in physical activity and nutrition that have fueled the obesity epidemic' (Centers for Disease Control and Prevention 2008).

How the conclusion of a general and widespread anti-food bias was arrived at is not made clear in *Diet Nation* and no evidence is offered for it. The authors also make no mention of the large research literatures devoted to understanding and changing people's physical activity choices and behaviours as well as research into promoting physical activity at the community level. Basham, Gori and Luik have apparently not read or listened to the constant moaning about a couch potato generation of children by academics, journalists and politicians in all Western countries over the last ten years. I have kept a file of scientific and newspaper articles, now numbering in the hundreds, in which the physical laziness of children and adults is endlessly repeated and simply taken for granted. Basham, Gori and Luik are apparently not aware of the hundreds of mass-participation physical activity interventions being trialed and implemented in communities all over the world. They also make the argument that the anti-food bias of obesity crusaders is evident from their preoccupation only with Western food environments, while neglecting the influence of the built environment on physical activity levels. This is a remarkably inaccurate proposition for a book that, on certain issues, is forensic in its treatment of the relevant literature. On the contrary, there is a great deal of research into both the effect of the built environment on physical activity levels as well as ways in which the built environment might be manipulated to increase physical activity (for example Burdette and Whitaker 2004; Frank, Andresen and Schmid 2004; Frank, Engelke and Schmid 2003; Wen, Orr, Millett and Rissel 2006). None of this is discussed in *Diet Nation*. Instead, obesity crusaders are painted as insufferable and puritanical food-hating kill-joys: 'The obesity crusaders' battle cry carries the implicit message that food consumption is a necessary evil. Eating is something that, regrettably, we must do in order for us to be able to do everything else in our lives' (Basham, Gori and Luik 2006: 202).

In passing, the authors of *Diet Nation* are far from the only obesity sceptics to assert that obesity medicine and science or public health authorities are driven by a mean-spirited hatred of people's pleasure (for another example see Fitzpatrick 2006). Whatever else might be said about this claim, I am not aware of any attempt to justify it. In fact, it is difficult to know how statements of this kind could ever be substantiated and it is self-evident, I think, that the targets of the accusation would deny it. In other words, the idea that the proponents of the obesity epidemic, as a class of people, see food as a 'necessary evil' is nothing more than a petty moral slur.

With respect to physical activity, *Diet Nation* mostly only asserts that Westerners are doing less of it. A small number of sources are quoted and, as with *AEOM*, the authors seize uncritically on a few slender pieces of evidence. Having conceded that it is very difficult to know whether or by how much population physical activity levels have varied over time (see Basham, Gori and Luik 2006: 130), Basham, Gori and Luik then go on to make the bewildering claim that 'During the 1980s and the 1990s, physical activity declined by 13 percent' (2006: 254). Neither the kind of physical activity, nor where in the world this statistic holds true is explained. Do they mean that all forms of physical activity declined by 13%? In all countries? For all sub-groups of people?

Despite there being nothing approaching consensus in the literature about the relative contributions of gluttony and sloth and despite the uncertainties that they themselves concede, the authors of *Diet Nation* are unequivocal in their conclusion: 'As has been detailed, contemporary weight gain is not the result of higher food consumption; rather it reflects a reduction in physical exertion' (Basham, Gori and Luik 2006: 253). It is worth mentioning that this is not a context-specific assertion. Basham, Gori and Luik apparently think this is true for the entire Western world and no concession to local variation of any kind is entertained. To my mind, this is an obvious example of the way depth of ideological commitment tends to encourage the speaker or writer to over-reach themselves, blinding them to the subtleties and contingencies of the subject at hand.

This point becomes even more striking in light of the book's final section that discusses at some length the limitations of observational epidemiology. Basham, Gori and Luik correctly point out that many of the claims made by alarmists, particularly those concerning the health risks of being overweight or obese, rest on statistical correlations between data of dubious reliability. They write:

> Even more perplexing is that statistical elaborations presented in most epidemiological studies are based on the assumption that the original data on which statistical analyses are performed are reliable and accurate, and provide objective measurements of real conditions. In fact, this assumption is wholly unwarranted, given that the original data are obtained through manifestly unreliable individual recalls that guess compositions and amounts of lifetime diets, or levels of exposure to possible hazards. Thus, for many epidemiological studies, the inescapable conclusion is that the statistical elaborations offered are demonstrably figments of the imagination, and this holds true for studies that either may or may not support a particular issue, such as the obesity epidemic.
>
> (Basham, Gori and Luik 2006: 286–287)

This passage sums up a significant aspect of the critique of obesity as a looming health crisis. And while the authors have research into the health of effects of certain diets in mind here, the point also applies to studies concerned with the connections between body weight and morbidity/mortality. But if you live by the sword, you risk dying by the sword; this same critique applies to the research Basham, Gori and Luik cite to support their case that people are generally less active and that more sedentary living has serious health consequences. Physical activity research also relies largely on observational epidemiology and self-report data and the problems here are exactly the same as for dietary research. For example, in *Fat Politics* Oliver notes that it is difficult to be sure whether population physical activity levels are changing but notes:

> According to recent Gallup polls, over the past decades, the percentage of Americans who exercise has actually increased to more than twice the number from a generation ago. Studies of Americans' daily time usage indicate that the average number of minutes Americans spent in leisurely and discretionary physical activity increased from twenty-seven minutes per day in 1965 to forty-seven minutes per day in 1995.
>
> (2006: 150)

As Jan Wright and I attempted to demonstrate in *The Obesity Epidemic*, obesity research has not delivered anything approaching a clear answer to the perennial question of food versus physical activity. In fact, the intractable difficulties inherent in this question have caused some leading obesity researchers to suggest that we should just give up trying to answer it and get on with the job of fighting the war on fatness (for example, see Research Update 2009).

At the risk of the labouring the point, Basham, Gori and Luik attempt to support their physical activity thesis by pointing to research that shows that less people are employed in manual occupations in agriculture and industry. But this is just one of many examples where they have either not done their homework or just been highly selective in their choice of research studies. A number of studies have attempted to measure the effect of manual occupations on body weight and consistently found that people employed in non-manual jobs tend to be less over-weight and obese than manual workers (for example Gutiérrez-Fisac et al. 2002; Czernichow et al. 2009). As with most of the points I have raised in this section, it is not that I can prove that Basham, Gori and Luik are wrong, but rather that it is easy to show that their case is built on, at best, incomplete or, at worst, selective sources of evidence.

Two final aspects of *Diet Nation* are worth considering. First, while *AEOM* makes a few passing references to the issue of personal responsibility, for *Diet Nation* this is a primary concern. Basham, Gori and Luik argue that the obesity crusaders over-emphasise our corporate-driven food environment and de-emphasise physical activity because they have an ideological bias against the concept of personal responsibility. In turn, this bias grows from a public health mentality that sees policy as synonymous with regulation. Thus, the obesity cru-sader seeks to co-opt government by picking on easy targets for regulation such as the food industry:

> Nor does the explanation of obesity as a product of individual choice work as a foundation for the policy aspirations of the obesity crusader. This is because, if obesity is a problem brought about by something that individuals choose to do, rather than by something that is done to them by their environment, then it is much more difficult to justify involving the government in solving the problem.
>
> (Basham, Gori and Luik 2006: 131)

At this point it is important to at least remind readers that many of the peo-ple Basham, Gori and Luik label as 'obesity crusaders' criticise the so-called 'personal responsibility' approach to obesity not on philosophical grounds, but because, they argue, it has been tried and shown not to work. This certainly also seems to be the view of many obesity sceptics, including Gasser, Campos and Oliver. At the same time, as I will show in Chapter 7, there are many commen-tators, particularly in the social sciences, who argue that mainstream obesity science constantly emphasises personal responsibility. In addition, perhaps the dominant critique of the public health/health promotion approach to the obesity epidemic is the way it ignores the environments in which people live while imploring people to adopt so-called healthy lifestyle behaviours. Similar to the point I made about the extent to which Gasser, Campos and Oliver exag-gerate their difference from obesity alarmists, Basham, Gori and Luik seem unaware or prefer not to mention that their preoccupation with people's individ-ual physical activity choices is shared by a large section of the obesity research community.

Having first built and then incinerated their ideological straw man (i.e. obesity crusaders and their refusal to entertain the importance of personal responsibility),

Basham, Gori and Luik then offer us their prescription for dealing with obese people. They are careful to make clear that we really only need to be concerned with the extremely obese – they do not spell out where 'extreme' obesity cuts in – and that health authorities should leave the rest of us alone. But rather than trying to help extremely obese people, they recommend that the situation calls for tough love, or what they unapologetically call 'discrimination':

> To the extent that obesity may be a real problem, it is a problem for individuals. The taxpayers of this country [here they presumably mean Great Britain] should not be expected to take care of those individuals who simply refuse to take care of themselves.
>
> (Basham, Gori and Luik 2006: 260)

We have already seen how some obesity sceptics construct alarmists as a relatively small renegade group. Likewise here: in order to stigmatise obese people in this way Basham, Gori and Luik appear to have tried to make their target reassuringly small. For example, imagine if a policy of intentional body-weight based discrimination by employers, schools and insurers, and strongly endorsed in *Diet Nation*, applied to a large proportion of society:

> First, this policy [of discrimination against extremely obese people] would place the costs for being overweight squarely on individuals, giving them stronger incentives to slim down. Second, since most employers want a healthy workforce, it would give them an incentive to help employees control their weight, perhaps by restricting what is served in the company canteen, or offering exercise facilities. In 2002, Southwest Airlines initiated a policy of requesting that its largest passengers – those who require two seats on an aeroplane – purchase two tickets.
>
> (Basham, Gori and Luik 2006: 266)

This kind of formulation is anything but original and has been circulating around free-market and libertarian think tanks for some time. Take the following from the Canada-based Simon Fraser Institute:

> If governments decide to act, however, the best way to account for the costs the obese impose on society is to require these individuals to bear those costs that result from their decisions. This could be as simple as introducing health premiums scaled by the cost that individual's lifestyle choices imposes on others. A scaled premium not only solves the problem of an increased burden on all Canadians created by the few who may be able to choose otherwise, but also gives those who are obese a reason to lose the extra pounds . . . If governments insist on acting, for whatever reason, they must avoid the bad policies that are commonplace in the discussion today. The way to deal with the problem is clear: require those who can choose otherwise to bear the burden of the costs they impose on others.
>
> (Esmail and Brown 2005)

The final aspect of *Diet Nation* that deserves comment follows on from its focus on personal responsibility, but it also goes to the heart of my interest in the arguments that different obesity sceptics make. One of the most detailed sections of the book is its treatment of the debate surrounding food advertising. Focusing on various governmental reports that have recommended regulating food advertising to children, Basham, Gori and Luik show how expert panels have tended to be lazy in their consultations of relevant literature, guilty of framing the issue in self-serving ways and having preconceived opinions on the matter. In other words, Basham, Gori and Luik argue convincingly that the experts who governments have usually asked for advice about food advertising to children often have long histories as advocates against advertising. To some extent, this stands to reason; many people who involve themselves in research and advocacy do so initially because they have a pre-existing concern and desire to change some aspect of the world.

Basham, Gori and Luik also show how difficult it is to draw a direct causational line between food advertising, children's weight and short- or long-term health. Of course, this is something of a sleight of hand since, as they point out elsewhere in the book, a list of anything up to forty or fifty risk factors for obesity can be found in the research literature. What the authors do not mention is that while it is difficult to make a causational case against food advertising, if one limits oneself to published research it is just as difficult to build a causational case against any risk factor, no matter how apparently fundamental. After all, if each of the reported forty or fifty risk factors really does contribute to obesity, then the effect of each one is almost inevitably going to be small and inconsistent. For example, many obesity researchers readily concede that there is not even a conclusive empirical (as opposed to theoretical) case linking body weight with how much children eat and drink.

So, while Basham, Gori and Luik want their readers to believe that their arguments about food advertising are heretical and deal a devastating blow to the obesity crusade, nothing really could be further from the case. As with many obesity sceptics, one of their most important rhetorical manoeuvres is to exaggerate the extent to which they are overturning conventional wisdom and telling obesity alarmists something they do not already know. In other words, it is not so much the number or the quality of research papers that a given writer is able to marshal, what matters is the way evidence is framed and, just as important, what evidence is left out.

Diet Nation makes many contentious claims, from the centrality of physical activity in explaining the obesity epidemic to the assertion that the best way of helping extremely obese people is to discriminate against them. However, the most egregious of all is the accusation of bias amongst obesity crusaders, which is monotonously repeated throughout the book. For example, concerning a 2005 report by the Institute of Medicine into food advertising to children, we read:

> The disturbing thing is that, rather than a scientific report produced by means of a process that at least strives to be objective, we seem here to have a report

whose work is shaped by authors whose prior advocacy of a particular policy is not revealed.

(2005: 163)

And shortly after:

This is not to suggest that McGinnis, Kunkel or Dorr [authors of the Institute of Medicine report] are not entitled to their views about food advertising, obesity and children; it is simply to say that they did not approach their work without substantial bias, and that the reader was not informed of this bias.

(Institute of Medicine 2005: 164)

Although the profiles at the front of the book mention some of the organisations with which the authors are associated, at no stage does *Diet Nation* explain what preconceived ideas *its* authors brought to the issue of obesity. Without doing some independent research, the reader finishes the book none the wiser about the authors' long history of advocating for small government, personal responsibility and free markets. No explanation is offered as to how *these* biases have affected the book's conclusions. For example, the authors do not tell readers whether their research into obesity led them to believe that emphasising personal responsibility is a more prudent course of action compared to government regulation, or whether this was a bias they began with. Neither are readers asked to consider the fact that the authors have in the past written about a wide range of subjects – including election campaign finance, the wars in Iraq and Sri Lanka, smoking, illicit drugs and gambling – and on each occasion argued the same free-market libertarian line. No, the authors of *Diet Nation* have simply wrapped themselves in the flag of scientific rigour and objectivity, crossed their fingers and, it appears, hoped that no one would recognise their faces.

Before moving to the next section, I want to offer a final example of what can happen when the idea of the obesity epidemic is refracted and distorted through the lens of free-market thinking. Eric Finkelstein and Laurie Zuckerman's (2008) *The Fattening of America: How the Economy Makes Us Fat, If it Matters, and What to Do About It* is not, strictly speaking, a piece of obesity scepticism. In fact, for much of the book the authors tread the worn path of obesity alarmists before them. They write, '. . . researchers at the University of Illinois at Chicago have made a surprising new prediction: Due to increases in the prevalence of childhood obesity, today's children may not live as long as their parents' (Finkelstein and Zuckerman 2008: 5).

As we saw in Chapter 2, this is anything but a 'surprising' or 'new' prediction. Amazingly, the authors also seem either unaware or intent on obscuring the controversies surrounding body weight and American mortality (see Chapter 2):

In fact, according to one recent study, poor diet and physical inactivity may soon overtake tobacco as the leading cause of death in America. The study reported that the three leading causes of death were tobacco (435,000 deaths;

18.1% of total U.S. deaths), poor diet and physical inactivity (365,000 deaths; 15.2 percent), and alcohol consumption (85,000 deaths; 3.5 percent).

(Finkelstein and Zuckerman 2008: 10)

They also recycle the idea of ongoing and unbridled obesity rate increases:

> Regardless of terminology, even more alarming than the high prevalence is the rate at which excess weight is rising among America's youth. Government data reveals that the rate of overweight 6 to 11 year olds tripled from 4 percent to almost 19 percent during the past 30 years. (4) . . . WHO predicts that if current trends continue, the number of overweight or obese people will increase to 2.3 billion and the number of obese will almost double to 700 million by 2015.
>
> (Finkelstein and Zuckerman 2008: 13)

But there is a twist here. The authors are economists and, thanks to books like *Freakonomics* (Levitt and Dubner 2005), write in the recently popular field of behavioural economics. For the uninitiated, behavioural economics attempts to explain human decision making by using economic principles, particularly the idea of rational utility maximisation. In short, the golden rule here is that we always do things to maximise our own economic self-interest. Needless to say, Finkelstein and Zuckerman (2008) see body weight as an essentially economic matter. In part, this leads them to argue that, compared to decades ago, modern Americans eat more calories because high-calorie convenience foods have become cheaper relative to fruit and vegetables and modern Americans do less exercise because physical activity has become more expensive. This does not only mean that for many of us exercise is something for which we now have to pay money. It also means that in order to get regular exercise we need to give up doing other things that might earn us more money or that we simply enjoy more than exercise. In other words, there are, the argument goes, significant opportunity costs involved in being physically active.

The alert reader will see where this logic is heading. First, for Finkelstein and Zuckerman (2008), rising obesity is the result of unnecessary government intervention in free markets; food subsidies have made unhealthy foods too cheap and urban planning has made physical activity too expensive. Second, they also argue that whatever weight an adult happens to be is the product of their rational utility-maximising choices; an obese person is obese because they value the enjoyment of food more than they value the benefits of being thinner. And it is here where *The Fattening of America* begins to work its way towards scepticism. Having unequivocally made the case for seeing obesity as a looming health emergency, Finkelstein and Zuckerman say that there is nothing that collectively we should do about it, at least for adults. Why? 'The above discussion suggests that there are no obvious market failures that are responsible for the rise in obesity rates in the United States. Therefore, government intervention cannot be justified on these grounds' (Finkelstein and Zuckerman 2008: 115). In other words, the authors are saying that there is no evidence to suggest that, fat or thin, people are doing anything other than freely expressing their desires and choosing to be who they want to be. This is a curious idea on at least a couple of levels.

First, Finkelstein and Zuckerman (2008) offer very little explanation for why two people would place a different value on being thin. In the world of behavioural economics, there are no cultural conditions or social forces that influence people's choices. So, as opposed to Basham, Gori and Luik's insistence that people's food choices be seen as a matter of personal responsibility, Finkelstein and Zuckerman turn to genetics. Ergo, people are born with an in-built, genetically hardwired and personalised set of desires upon which they then spend the rest of their life acting. This exquisite example of cherry picking odd bits of science in order to bolster a pre-existing ideological position is asserted as if it were a straightforward fact. The authors simply neglect to mention that genetic explanations of dietary preference remain highly controversial. Their determination to explain obesity via the twin ideologies of free-market capitalism and genetics is also probably why the authors studiously avoid talk of social class and make no mention of the consistent research finding that richer women and girls are thinner than poorer women across the Western world. The idea that anyone's choices might be constrained or shaped by structural disadvantage simply has no place here.

Second, in the world of utility-maximising individuals, there is no such thing as internal conflict. Thus, for Finkelstein and Zuckerman (2008), people who love their food *and* want to be thin do not exist. Likewise, the person who diets, perhaps yo-yoing between weights, struggling with their desires or hating themselves when the pleasure of food gets the better of them does not exist. And as for anyone who is fat but wants to be thin, well, they are simply in denial about their true self. After all, if they really did want to be thin they would just get up off the couch and be thin.

While not sounding much like a flesh-and-blood human, the cost-benefit analysis machine-person of behavioural economic theory does exist for a reason: to defend the interests of commerce. Nothing should be done to fight obesity that would inconvenience business, except, perhaps, in schools. The circularity of this formulation should be obvious. We start with a theory derived from observations in the world of commerce that is then universalised to explain not just an aspect of people's behaviour, but human nature itself. This vision of human nature then bounces back from whence it came: the behaviour of commerce is beyond criticism because, unsurprisingly, it is held to be consistent with human nature. People buy what they want to buy, eat what they want to eat and move when and as much as they want to move.

In the end, the reader of *The Fattening of America* is offered an extraordinarily counter-intuitive conclusion: obesity is a huge public health crisis, but nobody (other than meddling governments) is to blame and nothing should be done; people should not be encouraged to be more responsible and corporations should not be forced to change their behaviour. For Finkelstein and Zuckerman, the challenge that faces us is defending business from the unnecessary and unwise government interventions that the obesity lobby proposes. Rather than more medical assistance for people with obesity-related disease, we should provide less support, and particularly less generous health insurance, because this support artificially reduces the costs of being fat. If the costs of being fat were higher then fewer people would get fat. Employers should be allowed to discriminate against fat people because it makes good economic sense to do so. After all, Finkelstein and Zuckerman (2008) say, fat people are absent from work more often and are less productive than thin people (for example, see Finkelstein and Zuckerman 2008: 96 and 192–193).

At the beginning of this chapter I said that I was interested in the way ideological biases shape what people think, believe and advocate. *The Fattening of America*, like *Diet Nation*, is a superb example of ideology in action. But it is also interesting to see the way two sets of authors, ostensibly coming at the obesity epidemic with closely aligned free-market allegiances, make such different arguments about key issues. For example, *The Fattening of America* and *Diet Nation* completely disagree about the seriousness of rising obesity levels. They also differ sharply on questions of morality and personal responsibility; the authors of *Diet Nation* want to emphasise personal responsibility because this exonerates the behaviour of corporations, while the authors of *The Fattening of America* want to silence talk of morality since it tends to complicate and undermine their dry economic faith in a world populated by rational individuals making rational choices based on the relative costs of goods and services. And while *Diet Nation* wants to protect big business on the grounds that there is no obesity crisis, the authors of *The Fattening of America* apparently believe that a crisis exists but that trying to do anything would interfere with the workings of the market and make the situation worse.

The hard men

So far we have seen two broad types of empirical sceptics: the 'truth tellers' who contrast themselves with what they see as the corrupt and incompetent 'health establishment' and another group that, in different ways, sees the obesity epidemic as an attack on freedom and free markets. The final sub-group, the 'hard men', make many of the same arguments about science and freedom, but with a twist. Rather than liars, con men and socialists, the hard men are hunting a different enemy altogether.

In 2005 the Oxford-based Social Issues Research Centre (SIRC) published *Obesity and the Facts: An analysis of data from the Health Survey for England 2003*. As with Gaesser, Campos and Oliver, the use of the word 'facts' boldly announces that the authors will brandish the truth against the forces of ignorance and bias.

Purporting to analyse published data from the United Kingdom's Department of Health, *Obesity and the Facts* (SIRC 2005) argues that childhood body weights in the United Kingdom changed very little between the years 1993 and 2003. It claims that health authorities have erred by using outdated childhood weight distribution curves which are based only on United Kingdom data and fail to take into account the upward secular trend in children's height. If, instead, more recently published distribution curves based on international data are used, *Obesity and the*

Facts argues that the idea of a childhood obesity crisis begins to look fanciful. For example, it claims that:

> The average weight of boys aged 3–15 years in 1995 was 32.0kg. In 2003 it was 31.9kg. For girls the figures were 32.0kg and 32.4 kg respectively.
>
> The average 15 year old boy weighed 60.7kg in 2003, compared with 58.8kg in 1995. For 15 year old girls the figures were 58.9kg and 58.5kg respectively.
>
> (SIRC 2005: 2)

The authors write:

> We can conclude from these figures that there have been no significant changes in the average weights of children over nearly a decade. This can be taken as evidence that there has been no 'epidemic' of weight gain, since an epidemic would certainly have affected average weights.
>
> (SIRC 2005: 3)

And later:

> With these data before us, it is hard to understand why so much of the emphasis and related investment in public policy initiatives to tackle obesity has been directed towards children and young people – attacks on consumption of 'junk food', proposed restrictions on advertising of 'sugary fatty foods' – when the problems are most evident in older generations.
>
> (SIRC 2005: 9)

I was initially curious about *Obesity and the Facts* given its potential usefulness for my own research and advocacy. But I was also curious. Who or what is SIRC? The centre's web page says, 'SIRC is an independent, not-for-profit organisation based in Oxford, UK. We conduct research on a wide range of social topics and combine robust qualitative and quantitative methods with innovative analysis and thinking' (www.sirc.org).

While this seems unremarkable enough, clicking 'About SIRC' reveals the following:

> SIRC aims to provide a balanced, calm and thoughtful perspective on social issues, promoting open and rational debates based on evidence rather than ideology. In pursuit of this balanced perspective, SIRC conducts research on positive aspects of social behaviour as well as the more problematic aspects that are the focus of most social-science research.
>
> (www.sirc.org/about/about.html)

Once again we have a group of writers who claim to be untouched by ideological bias. Notice also their claim to be 'balanced' and 'calm'. 'Balanced' seems predictable enough but what about 'calm'? Why do they feel the need to stress how calm they are?

Some readers will notice that the first named member of SIRC's 'Panel of Advisors' is Desmond Morris, the well-known zoologist whose most famous publication is perhaps *The Naked Ape* (1967). Morris was one of the founding figures of sociobiology, the scientific movement that emerged in the late 1960s and early 1970s and claimed to show that human behaviour, including gendered behaviour, was the result of Darwinian natural selection. Sociobiologists positioned their work as a critique of social constructionist and feminist social science because, they claimed, gendered behaviour was predominantly 'natural', rather than the product of culture. Morris's fellow members on SIRC's panel include anthropologists Robin Fox and Lionel Tiger, whose 1980s and 1990s work articulated the extremes of biological determinism, famously lamenting that contraception has wounded men's 'natural' position at the head of kinship groups by artificially liberating women from men's control (in particular, see Tiger's relatively recent 1999 book, *The Decline of Males*). The centre's co-directors include Kate Fox, Robin Fox's daughter, and Peter Marsh, an occasional co-author with Desmond Morris.

In short, members of SIRC include authors of some of the most misguided and repugnant social science ever written. In particular, there could be few writers who have done more than Desmond Morris to popularise the idea that gender relations and social inequality are biologically determined and that attempts to bring about social change are both dangerous and futile.

The meaning behind SIRC's claims to offer 'a balanced, calm and thoughtful perspective on social issues' and to conduct research 'on positive aspects of social behaviour as well as the more problematic aspects that are the focus of most social-science research' is now more clear. Much of the research listed on SIRC's web pages takes a decidedly celebratory attitude to everyday life. For example, feminist scholars who have criticised the dominance of male sports in Western culture will be interested in SIRC's commissioned report *The Impact of Sport on the Workplace* (SIRC 2006a). The report's cover shows attractive young people in business dress, smiling and clapping as they presumably watch sport on an out-of-shot screen. And contrary to commentators who have bemoaned the money, attention and cultural kudos given to elite sports people, *The Impact of Sport on the Workplace* recommends that employers create more opportunities for employees to watch, celebrate and talk about elite sport.

The work of SIRC represents a particular kind of critique of academic social science. Its members are against what they see as the undue influence of non-rational, evidence-free, ideological academic feminism and the carping of university-based social scientists. Their view is that our social worlds are, to a large extent, given to us by our biological and cultural histories and that these should be judiciously respected, celebrated and preserved. As their self-description makes clear, they see themselves as a sober, scientific, objective voice in a culture preoccupied with risk and fear and inclined to believe the worst.

So, while SIRC's apparently one-off foray into obesity makes no mention of their social science enemies, it is consistent with their self-styling as muscular, unflinching opponents of a whining and timid academic mainstream. SIRC's target is not so much medicine or the enemies of capitalism, but a widespread propensity to believe things are worse than they are. As far as the actual substance of their critique goes, the idea that childhood obesity rates have been hugely exaggerated is one that I am inclined to support, although I am not as confident that they have discovered the 'facts' about obesity. *Obesity and the Facts* claims that its definitions for childhood obesity are 'less arbitrary' than other definitions, while 'Fattened Statistics', a SIRC (2006b) media release on the subject, suggests that their estimate represents the 'real' level of childhood obesity. And yet, *all* definitions of obesity are arbitrary, and this is particularly true for children. If 'obesity' means a level of body fatness that leads unequivocally to poorer short- or long-term health, we do not have anything approaching a scientific definition of obesity for children. In fact, BMI cut-off points, whether those endorsed by SIRC or anyone else, are generated from assumptions about rates of childhood growth not health risk. This issue is either obscured or not understood by the authors of *Obesity and the Facts*. The fact that their definition of obesity produces a lower prevalence rate is completely devoid of scientific significance unless it can be shown that their definition is more valid (i.e. more predictive of health risk). This is not even attempted.

Obesity and the Facts eventually argues that because childhood obesity prevalence is lower than adult prevalence, public policy should focus on adults. This apparent endorsement of the war on fatness raises doubts, at least in my mind, about the depth of SIRC's interest in obesity. Why would they bother to make this one narrow contribution to debate about obesity and then move back to their more familiar social science terrain? My guess is that, like all ideologues, SIRC is in the business of casting around for issues through which their existing world views can be prosecuted. In other words, despite the title of their report, the 'facts' about obesity are scarcely the point of the exercise.

By way of a final example, I turn to the 2005 edited volume *Panic Nation: Unpicking the Myths We're Told about Food and Health* (Feldman and Marks 2005). Edited by an anaesthetist (Stanley Feldman) and clinical bio-chemist (Vincent Marks), *Panic Nation* consists of thirty myth-busting chapters across a wide range of medical and health controversies.

The volume opens with a portrait of Peraclesus (1493–1541), the 'father of modern toxicology', and proceeds in a similar and unfailingly self-serious tone to take the sword to what the editors see as the trendy and dim-witted health and medical myths of the modern age. The consistent line of the thirty chapters is that pressure groups and bad scientists have managed to grossly exaggerate the health risks of things like salt, sugar, cholesterol, fast food and passive smoking, as well as pseudo-conditions like repetitive strain injury and stress-related illness. These same misguided groups have championed a wide range of useless, expensive and faddish pills, potions and interventions like food labelling, commercially available vitamins and minerals, complementary medicine, organic food and breast cancer screening. They are also responsible for scurrilously impugning the reputation of standard medical interventions like hormone replacement therapy and child immunisation. By contrast, the chapters are exclusively pro-business; they give a clean bill of health to food additives, pesticides and genetically modified food. Likewise, the air we breathe has never been cleaner and there really is nothing to worry about from mad cow disease.

Taken together, *Panic Nation* asks us to put our trust in two institutions: private enterprise and mainstream scientific (as opposed to fringe and alternative) medicine. Our enemies are radical environmentalists, new agists, vegetarians, feminists and health and fitness nuts, or what the editors collectively call 'pressure groups'. The tone of the book is perfectly captured in Marks's chapter on 'healthy eating'. Here, the self-image of the book's authors as sage purveyors of scientific, time-honoured truths immune to the fashions and hysterias of the day is all but spelt out:

> The famous food pyramid, introduced to simplify the healthy eating message and based upon 1980s dogma, is already outmoded and incorrect. What is the advice on healthy eating today? I believe that, as in the past, we should eat a variety of different foods from the dairy, grocer, baker, fruiterer, greengrocer and vintner, and somewhat less frequently from the fishmonger and butcher, in portion sizes and total quantity that ensures proper growth in children and the maintenance of a body mass index of around 20–25 in young adults and 23–27 in older adults. This coupled with moderate daily exercise, involves a lifestyle that becomes easier to practice once one understands the reason why it is good for one's health.
>
> (Marks 2005a: 50–51)

It is difficult to know whether Marks's use of words like 'fruiterer', 'vintner' and 'fishmonger' are quaintly and innocently anachronistic or assertively nostalgic and conservative. I heard Vincent Marks discussing *Panic Nation* on the radio around the time of its release. He was clearly a man of considerable age and spoke with the patrician tones we might stereotypically expect of a man who first studied medicine at Oxford in the late 1940s. His message concerning the value of traditional wisdom ('as in the past') and moderation (as opposed to trendy fanaticism) in all things, though, is unmistakable.

Marks's chapter on obesity claims that the risks of obesity have been exaggerated, marshalling similar arguments as the ones made by other authors discussed in this chapter. He writes:

> As people get older, there is population shift from the lower to the upper half of this range. Plumpness in late-middle and old age, especially in women, is not as great a health risk as it is in young and middle-aged adults – indeed it is often an advantage for longevity. Plumpness in childhood, often called 'puppy fat', is common, and the evidence linking it to adult obesity is conflicting. What is certain, though, is that gross obesity is a real hazard but, in spite of what one reads in the media, this is rare and normally due to genetic and metabolic defects.
>
> (Marks 2005b: 54–55)

As we have seen, for Gaesser, Campos and Oliver, obesity hysteria is the fault of the 'health establishment', by which I take them to mean mainstream obesity researchers and health officials. But Marks and his co-contributors in *Panic Nation* take an opposite view. They clearly think there is nothing wrong with mainstream obesity science and medicine. In fact, Marks concludes his chapter on obesity by saying that advances in medical knowledge are the only 'genuine hope' (Marks 2005b: 60) that obese people have.

In a later chapter, rather than science Feldman (2005) blames 'the media' for spreading misinformation about fatness and 'pressure groups' for popularising the concept of 'junk food'. Echoing the free market sceptics, Feldman can barely conceal his anger, describing the term 'junk food' as an 'oxymoron' (2005: 61). For the kind of writers both Marks and Feldman appear to be, this seems an odd argument. With their decidedly 'old school' hat on, they clearly have no time for what is often called 'relativism'; the idea that all judgements are relative and that there is no such thing as absolute scientific truth. And yet, when it comes to food, Feldman suddenly morphs from old-fashioned curmudgeon into card-carrying new-age postmodernist, demanding that the idea of junk food is a myth, that all foods are equally valid and that it is unfair to see some foods as better than others. Feldman does this in order to defend the makers of fast food from their 'trendy' 'pressure group' enemies.

Panic Nation is also cooler about the need for more physical activity than other empirical sceptics. In his chapter on 'Sports and exercise', Michael Aichroth says that 'Sport is a double-edged sword' and emphasises the risks and costs of too much exercise (2005: 268). His recommendation is that a little brisk walking every day is all that is needed to counter the negative effects of an unhealthy lifestyle. Meanwhile, he criticises pressure groups for over-selling the benefits of 'excessive' exercise, especially organised sport.

Taken together, the eighteen male contributors to *Panic Nation* craft their scepticism out of an allegiance to mainstream, 'respectable' medical science and their opposition to single-issue groups and the enemies of business. The book's overwhelming impression is of plaintive wish to go back to a time when doctors, scientists and businessmen enjoyed the unquestioning admiration they deserve – a time unsullied by the suspicions of feminists, environmentalists and all the other trendy enemies of science and reason. While for Gaesser, Campos and Oliver obesity science's problem exists inside the tent, for the authors of *Panic Nation* the problem is the barbarians outside.

We are only part of the way through this guided tour of obesity scepticism, but already we have a bewildering array of opinions from which to choose. Already we can see how the biases of the speaker predispose them to believe certain things. However, it is also particularly instructive, I think, to notice the way empirical sceptics all attempt to obliterate inconvenient uncertainty so the truth can be claimed as self-evident. And if the truth is self-evident then one's enemies must be mad, bad or just not very clever. In fact, what is consistent amongst the sceptics described in this chapter is not just their conspicuous self-styling as defenders of the truth, but the moral failings they attribute to their enemies. It is not simply that proponents of the obesity epidemic have been wrong. No, their crimes are much more serious than that, ranging from wilful ignorance and irresponsibility to bald-faced corruption. And as Chapter 7 shows, this is scarcely the half of it.

7   Power and theory
The 'ideological sceptics'

I now turn to a strain of scepticism that is less concerned with the science of the obesity epidemic and more with its philosophical, ethical and political dimensions. Rather than attempting to argue against obesity science by offering an assessment of the evidence, these authors tend to rely on the work of the empirical sceptics in order to mount other kinds of arguments about the causes and effects of the war on fatness. Below the buzz of scientific claim and counter-claim, they see deeper ideological forces at work.

From the start, it is important to emphasise that there is nothing illegitimate about accepting the work of other scholars and writers and using it for ones own purposes. Building on the insights of others is one of the primary ways in which most of us try to understand the world and it would be difficult to see how anyone could speak or write about any subject without first taking certain ideas for granted.

But as with Chapter 6, I am interested in *which* things people take for granted and why they do this. In other words, what are the politics of the knowledge claims they make? We have just seen how obesity sceptics who see themselves as the defenders of free enterprise dogmatically cling to the much-disputed idea that food consumption has played no significant role in rising rates of obesity. Likewise, in this chapter I examine how and why a second group of sceptics make specific choices about what they appear to believe.

I will call this second group 'ideological sceptics', although a similar caveat to the one I offered in Chapter 6 applies. I hope it is abundantly clear to readers that I see empirical sceptics as anything but ideologically neutral. In the same way, I do not use the term 'ideological sceptics' because I think these writers are any more or less ideologically committed or compromised. Rather, I want to draw attention to the way ideological sceptics justify their critiques of the obesity epidemic primarily in terms of particular political and ideological struggles.

I accept that in some cases my distinction between empirical and ideological sceptics will seem artificial and stretched. However, in my defence I would stand by the claim that all of the empirical sceptics discussed in Chapter 6 situate their arguments primarily within an assessment of obesity science. With this as their rhetorical foundation, they then ask us to accept their more ideologically and politically loaded arguments. In other words, as disingenuous or mistaken as I might sometimes suspect them to be, their strategy is science first, politics second. In this respect ideological sceptics are quite different; although they often allude briefly to obesity science, they are primarily interested in the underlying cultural and social biases that brought the obesity epidemic into being and, most importantly, shape what they see as its damaging effects in the world.

Whether or not the reader accepts this distinction, the sceptics I discuss in this chapter make very different, sometimes diametrically opposed arguments to the ones we have just seen. In fact, the picture that I hope to have created through this chapter and the previous chapter is of a mosaic of sceptics, idiosyncratic in their views and ideas, with almost nothing that is common to them all save for their hostility to the war on fatness. Ultimately, I will leave it to readers to decide whether the cumulative work of sceptics adds up to a compelling alternative to the alarmist rhetoric of the obesity mainstream. However, I would want to at least remind readers of the central point Jan Wright and I made in *The Obesity Epidemic* (Gard and Wright 2005): obesity science – the field of study that gave us the idea of an obesity epidemic in the first place – is a vast, confused and confusing collection of opposing and apparently irreconcilable theories and ideas. There is no single coherent voice here either.

Ideological foundations

Ideological scepticism rests on one of two – often both – sets of received ideas. The first of these is what is generally known as the feminist critique of science. Here, science and, by extension, modern medicine are seen as institutions that embody a range of biases, including male over female, Western over non-Western, white over non-white, rich over poor, heterosexual over non-heterosexual, quantitative over qualitative and mind over body. Already I am on shaky ground because feminist writing about science comprises a huge and diverse literature. However, my point is that the feminist critique of science and medicine is the primary intellectual well from which some ideological sceptics draw and, as we will see, determines the ways they are able to address the general question of how we should understand the obesity epidemic.

I want to stress here that the influence of the feminist critique of science is not limited to explorations of sexism in the practice or epistemology of science or the effects of science on girls and women, important as these dimensions are. Just as significant has been the feminist critique of science's attempts to see itself as purely objective, impersonal, valuing the supposed certainty of mathematical quantities and statistics, distrustful (and even afraid) of the variability and unpredictability of human bodies and inclined to (often mistakenly) see and/or impose order on the subjects of its enquiry. It is not simply that the feminist critique accuses science and medicine of being just another cog in the general and pervasively sexist machinery that constitute Western societies. Rather, science and medicine are singled out for being bastions of particular kinds of values and practices. Rather than merely mirrors to society, they are powerful forces that shape and, in some cases, mis-shape our world. In short, when I talk about the feminist critique of science, I am alluding not to a single premise, but a collection of ideas. My claim is that while these ideas are, in themselves, diverse and distinguishable from each other, they share a common ancestry.

The second set of received ideas that shapes the work of ideological sceptics is what I will call the 'critique of neo-liberalism'. Once again, in making this claim I have strayed into a vast scholarly minefield in which the existence, meaning, origins and effects of neo-liberalism are all hotly debated. Balanced against this complexity is the straightforward observation that ideological sceptics are in the business of taking up and applying the critique of neo-liberalism rather than being its authors.

In their anti neo-liberal vein, ideological sceptics see Western democracies as places in which citizens are under sustained rhetorical, social, moral, economic and political pressure to conduct themselves in certain ways. In particular, the modern neo-liberal citizen is expected to monitor even their most personal and intimate behaviours in order to contribute to the goals of the neo-liberal state and its institutions. In the critique of neo-liberalism these goals are taken to include the expression of free markets, economic growth and efficiency, individual self-reliance, homogenisation, consumer choice, predictability, control and a compliant, docile citizenry. While the goals of the neo-liberal state tend to be determined centrally, their enactment involves us all in the deepest nooks and crannies of our everyday lives. Some readers will be aware that this line of thinking owes much to the writing of the French intellectual Michel Foucault (for an extended discussion of this work see Harwood 2009), work that has been applied and reworked in a range of fields, but particularly in public health and health policy (for example, see Lupton 1995; Howell and Ingham 2001; Vander Schee 2008).

There are clear links between the feminist critique of science and the critique of neo-liberalism. Perhaps most pertinent to the discussion below is the attention authors working in both of these traditions pay to measurability, predictability and control in both the scientific and neo-liberal enterprise. My sense is that we can draw two conclusions about these areas of overlap. First, they make it easy, although not inevitable, for followers of one set of ideas to go along with the other. Second, however, they set the scene for furious agreement between scholars. In other words, we have the pre-conditions for group-think, so that important inconsistencies between the analyses of different writers are more likely to be ignored or glossed over.

My guess is that some readers will already assume my intentions towards these intellectual traditions are hostile. This is very far from the truth. The feminist critique of science is probably the most important foundation upon which I have built my intellectual life. I have no intention of disowning this legacy now. And although I offer a more complete account of my own position as an obesity sceptic in Chapter 8, it will soon become clear that my own thinking has much in common with the critics of neo-liberalism. It would be dishonest of me not to acknowledge this. I know and have worked with many of the writers cited here – a point that adds an extra layer of trepidation to the business of comparing, contrasting and, in some cases, evaluating this work. Suffice to say that in this chapter, as with the rest of this book, my purpose has been to pursue a robust and rational understanding of the obesity epidemic in a respectful and constructive manner.

Accepting fatness

For the uninitiated, the sheer existence of something called 'fat acceptance' can be something of a puzzle. In my experience, many people struggle to see or accept that there might be anything positive to say about being fat or that fat people might constitute a distinct group with a legitimate political agenda. However, writers and activists working within what has become known as the 'fat acceptance movement' have been challenging discrimination against fat people for at least forty years. That the creativity and talent of the movement's past and present leaders is not better known is surely evidence that prejudice against fat people remains pervasive.

Fat acceptance pre-dates the recent upsurge in interest about obesity by decades. In this sense, its activists and writers do not fit my post-2000 definition of obesity sceptics. However, their influence as an oppositional voice is ongoing and the arguments they have made are still being recycled today. Fat acceptance scholars and activists remain on the frontline of resistance to mainstream obesity rhetoric.

Early contributors to the movement, such as Louderback (1970), were amongst the first to argue that good health and fatness were not incompatible. Long before contemporary obesity sceptics, the fat acceptance movement, particularly in North America, argued that obesity science and medicine's treatment of fat people was not only flawed, but oppressive, particularly to women. Drawing directly on 1960s and 1970s feminism, fat activists blamed patriarchal psychologists, patriarchal researchers and patriarchal doctors for unfairly demonising fatness and pathologising the female body (for a retrospective discussion of this movement see the essays in Fallon, Katsman and Wooley 1994). Early feminist critiques of science were crucial here, adding intellectual momentum to more visceral political concerns. Fat activists used this literature selectively and for their own purposes, something they also did with the still only emerging science of fatness.

For example, many of the early feminist critics of science worked tirelessly to show that biology was not destiny and that male scientists had been wrong to conclude that there was some stable, universal and natural expression of masculinity and femininity, rendering others unnatural. Fat acceptance writers took up these arguments with gusto, claiming that dominant ideas about female appearance and behaviour were, likewise, patriarchal constructions designed to control and oppress women. Interestingly, though, when it came to body weight itself, the fat acceptance literature was almost uniform in its acceptance that biology *is* destiny. Looking back over more than a decade of fat activism in the edited volume *Shadow on a Tightrope: Writings by Women on Fat Oppression*, Vivian Mayer (1983) claimed that biology, not eating habits, is the main cause of fatness, that the health problems of fat people are caused by self-hatred, stress and chronic dieting, that dieting is bad for your health and that food binges are a natural response to dieting. She even generalised that the desire to please men is at the centre of women's self-hatred and weight problems. All this was done while citing, it appears, just enough scientific research to give these ideas an air of scientific credibility. Regardless of what one is inclined to make of Mayer's claims, it needs to be stressed that while the genetic contribution to both individual and population obesity levels is not well understood today, even less was known in the 1970s and 1980s.

The idea that fat people are the product of their genes proved irresistible to many fat acceptance writers and it was regularly offered to readers as if it were an established scientific fact. Contributing to the 1989 volume *Fat Oppression and Psychotherapy: A Feminist Perspective*, Goodman writes:

> We can no more be expected to change the fact that we're fat than to be expected to change the color of our skin. Granted, there are people who overeat, but it is now a proven fact in study after study that most fat people eat no more than their thin counterparts, and in some cases, it has been proven that they actually consume less. People who are fat from birth will always be fat.
>
> (1989: 13)

In the same volume, Tenzer is equally adamant:

> The fact is that fat people do not eat more than thin people, on the average. It has been difficult for the scientific community to concur that this is what the data supports because they have been brainwashed to believe that fat people have been gluttonous and dishonest about how much they actually eat.
>
> (1989: 43–44)

In her book *Fat – A Fate Worse Than Death? Women, Weight, and Appearance*, Thone repeats the claim:

> There are many in-depth studies that disprove the notion that large, fat, heavy – whatever you want to call them – people eat more than thin people. There are also many large, fat, heavy people who exercise regularly, wear stylish clothing, have good jobs, healthy relationships, travel widely, and generally live productive, rational, happy lives.
>
> (1997: 100)

The argument that fat people do not eat more than thin people rests on the well-documented empirical difficulties associated with precise measurements of caloric intake. What this literature points to is the complexity of human body weight and the challenges that researchers face when trying to control for all potentially relevant variables. Some studies support the idea that fat people eat more and some studies do not, but very few lead to firm conclusions either way. Claiming that over-eating –whatever this is taken to mean – plays little or no role in fatness is akin to arguing that a failure to show conclusively that car emissions exacerbate global warming or increase asthma levels proves that emissions are benign. Car emissions may or may not have these effects, but an ambiguous set of research findings does not settle the matter.

Some fat acceptance writers have approached the issue of culpability by referring directly to genetic control of body weight. In *Body Wars: Making Peace with Women's Bodies*, Maine writes that '. . . research shows that genetics account for at least 25%, and possibly as much as 70%, of the factors influencing weight, obesity is still considered sinful, a rejection of the highly valued ethics of self-denial and self-control, particularly for women' (2000: 19). Other writers, such as Chrisler, address the issue of personal responsibility by invoking the controversial scientific idea of a biological 'set point' body weight:

> Even referring to our clients as "overweight" suggests that there is a correct and obtainable weight and thus reinforces the stereotype of out of control people who are responsible for their weight. Recent physiological research has supported the existence of a genetic set point for weight and individual differences in metabolic activity.
>
> (1989: 35)

Why is this important? In her humorous and popular book *Fatso? Because you don't have to apologize for your size!*, Marilyn Wann (1998) invokes genetics to explain body weight and she selectively quotes a couple of research articles that suggest that fatness carries few health risks. As with the entire fat acceptance literature, my point here is not to tell other people what to write or how to conduct themselves. Authors like Wann scarcely need advice from me. Besides, *Fatso?* was written to be funny and thought provoking, not a summary of scientific evidence.

However, while some readers may have been inclined to agree with, say, the free market sceptics we met in Chapter 6, others may be more sympathetic to the cause of fat acceptance. What I want to suggest is that all sceptics are playing the same game – selecting and highlighting particular research findings and ignoring others – and our decision to go along with one group rather than another should take this into consideration. Certainly, free market thinkers like Basham, Gori and Luik would seize on fat acceptance's genetic arguments as an example of Western culture's flight from personal responsibility. For my part, while I understand why fat acceptance writers invoke genetics, I think they are mistaken to do so. This is not because I am worried about personal morality, but because one's freedom to eat and exercise as much or as little as one chooses is fundamental.

Cases of obesity caused by extreme metabolic disturbance or genetic inheritance are rare and more recent research into the genetics of body weight has not produced the simple answers that might once have seemed possible. In fact, researchers in this field readily concede that the genetics of body weight is still in its infancy (for example, see Kolata 2007). But putting all of this to one side, when fat acceptance writers invoke genetics they appear to misunderstand what researchers in this area actually do. Rather than being interested in whether they put on more weight given the same food intake, much more attention is given to why obese people appear to eat more food before they feel full. Put simply, the genetics of body weight focuses on appetite and satiety. Far from proving that fat people eat the same as anyone else, it generally assumes this to be false and then tries to discover genetic explanations for over-eating.

In my view, what matters is not whether a person chooses to become fat, but rather how much freedom society is prepared to afford people to do so. The idea that fat people eat more than other people is not, as Garrison and Levitsky (1993) suggest in *Fed Up! A Woman's Guide to Freedom from the Diet/Weight Prison*, a 'cultural myth'. If nothing else, arguments of this kind completely obscure the structural conditions that shape people's physical and social environments and, therefore, behaviour. They also play directly into the hands of those who would want to exonerate the behaviour of food corporations. For various reasons, some people do eat more than others, just as some people find exercise more painful, unpleasant, difficult, expensive or inaccessible. This fact does not make them morally inferior but, equally, it is does not turn their body weight, whatever it happens to be, into a predetermined genetic destiny. As incomplete and unsatisfactory as they sometimes are, narrow caloric (as opposed to genetic) explanations of body weight are not cultural myths.

New age feminism

When is 'the new age' not the new age? The answer for Jon Robison and Karen Carrier, authors of *The Spirit and Science of Holistic Health* (2004), is, as their book title suggests, when the spirit world is shown to be a scientific reality. Robison and Carrier write from the perspective of Health At Every Size (hereafter HAES), a coalition of nutrition and health workers and researchers who advocate against the importance of body weight as a marker for health and, most important of all, against conventional body weight-focused dieting. Robison, in particular, has been an ally of both fat acceptance and HAES and he writes prolifically about health.

If *Diet Nation* articulates the extremes of free market thinking applied to obesity, *The Spirit and Science of Holistic Health* (hereafter *SSHH*) stretches the feminist critique of science, crossed with obesity scepticism and (what at least to me feels like) new age spirituality to equally distant limits. There is no mincing words here. For Robison and Carrier, modern Western science and medicine are both patriarchal institutions:

> Traditional weight management approaches, *like all other aspects of Western health care*, emanate from the biomedical, reductionist paradigm, which is rooted in patriarchy and the oppression of women. On the surface it may look as though efforts to control body weight are simply based on a desire to make people "healthier." On closer examination, however, the disparate social emphasis on women regarding thinness, the emphasis on control over the body, and even the subtle messages that higher moral standing is obtained

through starving and denial of pleasurable eating are all perspectives that run directly parallel to the values of Epoch II and the Scientific Revolution.

(2004: 228, my emphasis)

The meaning of 'Epoch II' and 'the Scientific Revolution' deserve explanation. According to Robison and Carrier, humanity began in Epoch I, an idyllic matriarchal period in which there is no evidence of violence, war or anything other than people living in perfect harmony with the natural world: 'In these partnership societies there were no hierarchies of power and *no record of human on human violence*' (2004: 5, emphasis in original). This was followed by a patriarchal 'dominator epoch', Epoch II, in which patriarchal science emerged as the dominant human force. The scientific revolution of Epoch II gave us the technology to wage war, dominate and desecrate the natural world and enshrined rational reductionism and physical force over spiritual and holistic well-being. Robison and Carrier prophesy that we will soon move into 'Epoch III human soul' and that there are already signs that this transition is upon us. While it is never quite explained whether we are moving inevitably towards Epoch III or whether this is something we will have to work at, the authors certainly give the impression that, like end-of-days Christianity, Epoch III awaits and there is nothing much we can we can do about it. In fact, the religious overtones here are difficult to miss; Robison and Carrier (2004) assure us that the move toward Epoch III is part of the pre-determined evolution of the human soul.

Some readers will immediately hear echoes of Charles Reich's manifesto *The Greening of America* (1970) in Robison and Carrier's three epochs. Riding the wave of 1960s counter-culture ferment, Reich claimed that human culture was unfolding in three distinct phases: Consciousness I, a tranquil, rural past; Consciousness II, twentieth-century civilisation, its discontents, alienations and sicknesses; and Consciousness III, a future flowering of love, peace and boundless human potential for creativity and community. Both *The Greening of America* and *SSHH* suffer from the very obvious problem of failing to explain how we delineate aspects of Consciousness/Epoch II from Consciousness/Epoch III. For example, while Robison and Carrier (2004) claim that modern science and medicine have been the instruments of untold evil and oppression, their arguments for the kinder and healthier future that awaits are based on, yes, science. They apparently believe in the medical efficacy of prayer, healing at a distance and in 400 pages have not a single critical word to say about even the most fanciful forms of 'alternative' and 'complimentary' medicine. And yet their justification for these beliefs is intriguing. They believe in the power of positive thought to heal a person suffering a medical illness hundreds or thousands of kilometres away not on religious grounds, but because the *science* of chaos theory and the findings of quantum mechanics sanction these beliefs. Although a book written primarily for health promotion professionals – however, they claim, all health professionals should take heed – the authors write that the perverse and counter-intuitive world of quantum mechanics is *the* model for future understandings of health. So, although the wider scientific world still seems a very long way from a satisfactory 'theory of everything' synthesis between the physics of the micro and the macro, Robison and Carrier seem not the least bit daunted, going where no mainstream physicist would dare to tread:

> We learned from quantum physics that it is the relationship between sub-atomic particles that gives meaning to their existence. Similarly, in Holistic Health Promotion we emphasize that it is the relationships among the spiritual, biological, psychological, social and environmental dimensions of the human experience that are critical to a true understanding of health and healing.
>
> (2004: 171)

This confusion about when science is enemy and when it is friend is similar to the one we saw in the rhetoric of fat acceptance. Recall fat acceptance writers' damning criticisms of science and medicine's rank prejudice and biased research findings sitting right alongside their readiness to believe particular 'scientific facts' that supported their worldview. Likewise here; while it is theoretically possible that the tools of science might be used to create both the patriarchal, oppressive world we now inhabit as well as a future Utopia, how we tell when science is doing good or ill is not a detail with which Robison and Carrier concern themselves. They write that what they call 'holistic health promotion' will make '. . . the feminine value of compassion rather than the masculine value of control the guiding principle for health promotion' (Robison and Carrier 2004: 182). But surely one person's compassion is another person's control. When Robison and Carrier's patriarchal surgeon goes to work on the diseased tissue of a suffering patient, thus enacting all that is worst about the reductionist, violent, mechanistic Epoch II worldview, is she or he performing control or compassion?

Robison and Carrier's chaotic reasoning becomes yet more baroque as they turn their hand to obesity:

> There is no subject in health promotion more relevant to emerging Epoch III humanity than eating and weight. That may sound very strange! What do nutrition programming, weight loss classes, and body fat testing have to do with the decline of dominator societies and the arrival of the new consciousness? They have *everything* to do with it . . . Nothing has silenced the voices and energies of contemporary women more than dieting and body hatred.
>
> (2004: 227, emphasis in original)

This is a curious proposition. Robison and Carrier ask us to believe that Epoch II started about 4,500 years ago and the scientific revolution started about 400 years ago. As we saw above, it is this legacy, they argue, that has bequeathed our unhealthy bio-medical view of body weight. However, they then go on to suggest that worrying about body weight is actually a new phenomenon:

> The current American obsession with dieting and slimness is a cultural aberration. Throughout history, most cultures have regarded fatness as a sign

of success, health, and beauty. Less than one hundred years ago Americans equated body fat with affluence and higher socioeconomic status.

(Robison and Carrier 2004: 229)

If it is a defining element of 4,500 years of patriarchal Epoch II thinking, why has fat hatred only turned up in the last 100 years? If a more benign view of fatness will be the mark of the coming Epoch III, how could the celebration of fatness have also been the norm in Epoch II cultures? Is this island of fat hatred, on which we currently find ourselves marooned, an exception to the rule or business as usual? *SSHH* seems to say it is both.

Although it is credited with some significant achievements, there is a strong sense in *SSHH* that science can never win. In its more philosophical and theoretical moments, Robison and Carrier accuse science of being too much 'in the head' and not interested in the body. When science went into the body, largely via modern medicine, it was being too 'physicalist', at the expense of people's emotions. During those phases when science and medicine have been interested in emotion and behaviour, they are guilty of ignoring the 'spirit'.

Robison and Carrier begin their book by rejecting the 'new age' label, yet I struggle to see how *SSHH* could be categorised differently. But despite its idiosyncratic view of the cosmos and comical, half-baked philosophising, it returns almost precisely to the same core premise that is common to all obesity sceptics:

> Weight is irrelevant to health and mortality except at the most extreme levels of thinness and fatness . . . Fatness is associated with health benefits, including decreased death from some cancers, protection from osteoporosis, and improved recovery from respiratory diseases such as bronchitis and tuberculosis.
>
> (Robison and Carrier 2004: 242)

This assessment of body weight and health is perhaps a little more strident than other sceptics. The suggestion that weight is largely 'irrelevant' and the implication that there are clear-cut health benefits associated with significant adiposity are both highly optimistic readings of the research literature. But while some readers may question why I have even bothered to include it, my interest in a work like *SSHH* is that it is more a variation on a theme than a bizarre aberration. It rehearses many of the standard sceptical arguments, differing from other sceptics more on its credulity threshold; there seems almost no claim from both new age and conventional science that Robison and Carrier will not entertain. As an advocate for HAES and fat acceptance, Robison is regularly cited by popular and academic writers, suggesting that there are at least some people who share his ideas.

Neo-liberal bodies

Some readers will be aware that a vigorous debate about the pros and cons of what has come to be called the 'neo-liberal' orthodoxy has taken place in recent years. In its most widely understood form, the term 'neo-liberal' generally pertains to matters of economic and social policy. It is therefore most frequently subject matter for economists and political theorists and commentators. However, there exists a large theoretical and empirical social science literature that has attempted to understand how neo-liberal political and economic forces have shaped and are shaping life at a more personal day-to-day level, for example via our interactions with medicine, psychology, the media and education. Perhaps, more than anything else, this is a field of study that seeks to understand how our thinking about ourselves and our relationships with others are being affected by developments in the way we are governed and managed as citizens. Although this literature has not much concerned itself with body weight, there is a group of writers who have attempted to bring elements of the wider critique of neo-liberalism to bear on both the obesity epidemic and body weight-related matters.

The British academics John Evans and Emma Rich have been prominent here with their work in schools and with young women suffering from eating disorders (for example, Evans, Rich, Davies and Allwood 2005; Rich and Evans 2009). At the risk of over-simplification, this work argues that young people, particularly girls, find themselves under great pressure to conform and comply to a long list of educational and social expectations, while, at the same time, being stripped of a sense of control and autonomy. They write that life in today's schools can mean dealing with the twin forces of 'performativity' and 'managerialism', which combine to 'perfectly and terrifyingly represent the modernist quest for order, transparency and classification of consciousness prompted and moved by the premonition of inadequacy' (Evans, Rich, Davies and Allwood 2005: 3). In this formulation, the war on obesity is seen as symptomatic of a broader social environment in which we are also constantly instructed about how we should live our lives and the sense of failure we should feel if we do not measure up.

This is a similar set of arguments to those pursued by Christine Halse and colleagues (Halse 2009; Halse, Honey and Boughtwood 2007). Once again focusing on eating disorders, anxiety about body weight is understood as consistent with what they call the 'virtue discourses' of discipline, achievement and healthism (Halse, Anne Honey and Boughtwood 2007: 219; see also Zanker and Gard 2008 for an example of my own contribution to this literature which pursues a similar line of thought). So, eating disorders are seen as a kind of over-compliance with pervasive social pressures to be thin and healthy. But, more than this, the war on obesity also emerges from the neo-liberal impulse for control, conformity and predictability, while, at the same time, asking people to believe that they are in charge of their own destinies.

Other writers in this area have questioned the way anti-obesity-minded health policies have been articulated and enacted in ways that bear the hallmarks of neo-liberal thinking. For example, Fullager (2003, 2009) shows how public health campaigns appear to make dubious assumptions about how families live and the resources they have at their disposal to comply with public health messages. She also argues that physical activity health promotion tends to pitch a male-centric view of physical activity while overlooking the multiple pressures women are often under. As in Burrows's (2004, 2009) work in New Zealand, this line of argument has also been employed to think about culturally diverse contexts. In all of this work, be it focused on social class, gender, ethnicity or any marker of difference, these researchers argue that not only do neo-liberal health agendas embody hegemonic ideas about health and good citizenship, they also have the effect of blaming and holding people responsible for their failures to be the perfect neo-liberal citizen.

As a social scientist that has worked with these ideas and some of the scholars who use them, I am aware of at least two things. First, few writers working in this area are, at least to my knowledge, committed and unapologetic advocates for free-market capitalism. This will seem a trivial point to some readers, but I am talking here about a community of left-of-centre academics, including myself, for whom the idea that neo-liberal capitalism is the root of at least some of the evil in the world comes easily. My point, in other words, is that it is not a coincidence that, as a group, we have tended to see the obesity epidemic in similar anti-neo-liberal ways. Second and following on from this, there is a delicate line to tread between arguing, on the one hand, that the obesity epidemic is one of the somewhat unexpected and unwanted side effects of pervasive neo-liberal social forces and, on the other hand, that obesity alarmists are themselves the active and/ or deliberate agents of a neo-liberal agenda.

Let me explain what I mean by considering a few examples in which this second distinction, between unexpected side effects and the explicit motives of obesity alarmists, can become blurred. I begin with book *The 'Fat' Female Body*, a subtle and wide-ranging piece of scholarship by the Australian academic Samantha Murray (2008). Murray begins by taking issue with fat acceptance's (the author uses the alternative term 'size acceptance') faith in what she calls the 'liberal humanist' belief that the individual can change their reality. Here, Murray challenges an enduring line of thought within fat acceptance that stems from early feminist pro-fat therapy circles and, later, the self-help and pop psychology movements. In essence, this idea says that the secret to fat people living healthier and happier lives lies in changing the way they think about themselves.

It is worth pointing out that if *The 'Fat' Female Body* were simply about the politics and philosophy of fat acceptance then there would be no reason for discussing it in the context of obesity scepticism. Murray, though, makes it clear that she thinks we should doubt the idea of an obesity epidemic for a specific set of reasons. Like fat acceptance writers generally, Murray tends not to distinguish between, on the one hand, generalised and long-standing Western distaste for and anxiety about fatness and, on the other hand, the more recent surge in concern about obesity. For example, *The 'Fat' Female Body* begins with an intensely sexist quote from a 1924 *Journal of the American Medical Association* article in which a Dr James S. McLester clearly associates fatness with female ugliness and shallow character. But rather than this being an example of anachronistic medical opinion, Murray wants us to see this as consistent with modern views about obesity:

While medical narratives now speak in the authoritative language of apparently objective science, it is my contention that despite the 80 plus years that separate my research from the musings of McLester, what underpins the current 'panic' over 'obesity' in contemporary Western culture is a moral anxiety about the preservation of fixed gender identities and normative female sexuality and embodiment.

(2008: 3)

With perhaps the added interest in female sexuality, this is a feminist argument similar to the one commonly used in fat acceptance. In *Body Wars: Making Peace with Women's Bodies* Maine puts it this way:

By maintaining the status quo, Body Wars represent the clash between women's potential and their actual position in Western culture. As a society we are ambivalent and afraid of the implications of female power; better to keep women worried about their looks than to deal with the real issues of equality!

(2000: 3)

Over the course of the last chapter and a half we have heard many reasons for the existence of the obesity epidemic and here is another: the obesity epidemic exists to control women by keeping them anxious about their bodies as well as conventionally and conservatively heterosexual. Murray's argument is that it is not so much that health authorities care about people's health, but rather that they – and all of us, more generally – find the fat female body 'maddening' (Murray 2008: 5) and are made uncomfortable by it. Medical concern with obesity is not to make the fat body healthy, but to bring it under control.

In order to make this argument Murray coins the term 'disciplinary medicine' and it is here that we begin to see the merging of the feminist critique of science, dominant in fat acceptance and the work of writers like Robison and Carrier, and the critique of neo-liberalism. By 'disciplinary medicine' Murray means a form of medicine that wants to control and normalise, to make everyone look more or less the same, and – she goes further – to pass moral judgement on us all:

Moreover, as I will go on to show, medical narratives bring these normative discourses and assumptions under the ontological umbrella of the 'obesity epidemic'. It is here that anxieties about bodily difference are manifested as a 'moral panic': the threat this 'epidemic' poses is constituted by medical narratives not simply as endangering health, but as fraying the very (moral) fabric of society.

(2008: 15)

It is now clear that, unlike some of the empirical sceptics who blame small sections of the scientific and medical communities, Murray's target is the entire institution of medical science:

Medical science is preoccupied with measuring and quantifying bodies, establishing 'cut-off' points for bodies to slip over into pathology . . . The visibility of 'fatness' means that long before the results of any blood tests or ultrasounds or ECGS, the 'fat' body bears the mark not only as a *diseased body*, but a *moral failure* in medical narratives.

(2008: 26, emphasis in original)

The issue of moral failure is crucial here. As we saw above, there are times when Murray wants to argue that the war on obesity is 'underpinned' by a desire to make women feel bad about their bodies and to shame them into conformity. The previous quote, though, suggests something different: what we have is an unfortunate convergence of historical events whereby the recently launched war on fatness is being waged in Western societies already inclined to ascribe moral failure to the fat body. Either way, Murray makes a great deal of the idea that 'medical discourse' positions doctors and other health authorities as all-powerful and morally pure. For example, in a discussion about the 'clinical gaze', the process in which a medical expert surveys, inspects and makes judgements about the health of patients, Murray writes:

In other words, the function of the clinical gaze in these, and in fact, *in all clinical encounters* is, I contend, altogether different from the way in which society generally understands it, as a mode of pure scientific observation unfettered by personal bias, and thus possessed of an unquestionable authority. It is this understanding and concurrent functioning of the clinical gaze that preserves the authority of medical discourse and permits a widespread disciplinary operation.

(2008: 38, my emphasis)

At least to me, this seems an oddly old-fashioned view of people's attitudes toward medicine. There is, after all, a substantial literature focusing on the extent to which the modern medical consumer routinely questions the judgements of doctors, often suspecting them of all manner of biases, such as their choice of medications (for example, see Fitzpatrick 2001; Schlesinger 2002). From attention deficit hyperactivity disorder and immunisation to the treatment of depression, the Western world is awash in scepticism towards medical authority. In fact, the decline of medical authority in Western societies has been widely studied (Halpern 2004). Nonetheless, Murray takes a 1997 document concerning obesity from Australia's National Health and Medical Research Council as an example of the assumed moral superiority and unquestioned authority of institutional medicine and public health. Like hundreds of others, the document advocates a wide-ranging, some might say all-encompassing, approach to anti-obesity public health policy so that there would be few areas of our lives left unchanged if the authors had their way. Murray concludes:

The authority of the 'expert' and a tacit assumption about the moral superiority of people in "positions of influence" emerges here, whereby members of the community who occupy higher positions in the social hierarchy must become mouthpieces for the strategic plan, but more specifically, are rendered as incorruptible, infallible and paragons of virtue.

(2008: 30)

Murray seems to be saying that health authorities are positioning themselves as morally superior to the rest of us but that this is communicated by 'tacit assumption' (2008). Who is doing the assuming here? The writer of this document or the reader? Murray seems committed to a view of institutional medical and public health advocates who see themselves as morally superior. Is it Murray's pre-conceived idea about medicine that causes her to see tacit assumptions to this effect? It is certainly true, as I tried to show in the first half of this book, that advocates for the war on obesity regularly over-stretch themselves and constantly exaggerate the scale of the problem and the drastic measures needed to address it. It is also the case that a discourse of 'epidemic' and 'crisis' will inevitably breed its zealots. But it is quite another thing to assert that the entire anti-obesity agenda is a moral enterprise. I am at a loss to see how the rhetoric of the obesity epidemic, even at its most misguided, constructs health experts as 'infallible' or 'paragons of virtue' and an example of this does not spring readily to mind. In fact, obesity experts constantly concede the gaps in their knowledge, regularly arguing that we need to act despite these gaps. The only evidence Murray offers for her claim is her own assurance to readers that tacit assumptions really are lurking below the surface of the documents from which she quotes.

Why does Murray see such a powerful and, in fact, defining moral dimension to the obesity epidemic? We have already seen that she wants to convince readers that the war on fatness is designed to constrain and control women's bodies, identities and sexualities. However, my sense of it is that introducing this moral element also allows her to locate the obesity epidemic within the critique of neo-liberalism. This, in turn, is important because the research literature includes literally hundreds of examples in which experts describe the obesity epidemic as a problem of social and physical environments and categorically not an issue of individual culpability and personal morality. This presents the critic of neo-liberalism with a problem: how can you argue that obesity discourse is doing the bidding of small-government, free-enterprise, pro-personal responsibility ideology (*à la* Basham, Gori and Luik (2006) in *Diet Nation*) if obesity experts are actively calling for governments, not individuals, to solve the problem?

Murray's answer is to say that when medical authorities talk about changing the environment to make it easier for people to make healthy choices, what they are really doing is tacitly shifting responsibility back on to individuals:

. . . greater attention has been focused on environmental factors in order to explain rising 'obesity' rates such as the shift in mass food production and processing, resulting in an over-abundance of available food in developed countries, and more sedentary lifestyles at work and at home. The problem with this shift, as I will go on to discuss in greater detail, is that it reproduces the notion of individual (moral) responsibility: the belief that if only the individual would comply with health directives for 'health' (eating the 'right' foods, exercising more), 'obesity' could, and would, disappear.

(2008: 17–18)

Putting to one side the doubtful proposition that advocates of the healthy lifestyles message (eat better, exercise more) actually think it could ever bring about the complete eradication of obesity (no evidence for this is offered), Murray has created a perfect no-win situation here. If tomorrow Western health authorities collectively declared that the obesity epidemic was solely caused by the moral failings of individuals, they would be roundly condemned for victim blaming. However, in the examples that Murray offers, health authorities who explicitly focus on the environment are also accused of blaming individuals. Instead, she claims, when health authorities communicate their ideas about healthy living to the population they are, in fact, offering people only the illusion of choice; anti-obesity public health is a not about helping people to live happier, healthier, freer lives, but about social control and moral censure:

It is the function of disciplinary medicine, then, that connects the notions of self-policing, self-knowledge, self-transformation and moral responsibility. As I have explained, disciplinary medicine relies on the illusion of personal choice for all individuals, whereby each feels they freely choose to take up medical directives relating to 'healthy' lifestyles. In other words, the power of disciplinary medicine functions at a *tacit* level: the virtuous *appeal* of mastering one's own body in line with dominant health strategies *disguises* the disciplinary effect of medical discourse.

(Murray 2008: 22, emphasis in original)

What I think all this shows is that in order for the obesity epidemic to be cast as a form of oppression, in this case, against girls and women, a motive must be found. After all, it would not be enough to say that the anxiety and oppression felt by anyone was the regrettable but unintended consequence of an otherwise legitimate public health campaign since this situation would throw at least some of the responsibility back on those who claim to feel anxious and oppressed. Therefore, in order to make the case for oppression, Murray asks us to see disgust, condescension and the exercise of power, or, as she calls it, 'disciplinary medicine', embodied in health policies designed to create the mere illusion of a free society.

I have spent some time discussing *The 'Fat' Female Body* because it is emblematic of a particular form of ideological obesity scepticism that combines the feminist critique of science with the critique of neo-liberalism. Murray offers an ambitious and hugely thought-provoking analysis and my purpose here is not to dismiss it but to engage with what appear to be some of its most important claims. It is in many ways a more detailed and sophisticated elaboration of ideas that a number of other scholars, myself included, are exploring. My point, though, is to at least point out some of the potential pitfalls involved in applying a pre-existing theoretical lens to any social phenomenon.

Many close variations on Murray's arguments could be offered. Azzarito (2009) sees the obesity epidemic as an example of the way free-market thinking has invaded school education policy and, like Murray, detects a drive toward conformity: 'Campaigns against fatness concurrently contribute to the rise of "business-minded" schooling reform, academic analogues to "the bottom line (i.e., profit)" with "tendencies toward cultural homogenization" (Pinar 2004: 94), and the rise of the corporate curriculum' (2009: 184). And it is not just any kind of homogenisation at work here. Azzarito holds that the obesity epidemic emerges essentially from a white-skinned, Anglo-American world view. In short, the idea here is that the obesity epidemic and even dieting and physical exercise are, at their core, white discourses:

> . . . I contend that emerging school interventions, supposedly educationally based, are narrowly built upon the medicalization of young people's bod-ies, disavowing a socio-historical understanding of the construction of health and fitness discourses as embedded in whiteness, and implicitly function as a 'blaming the victim' approach . . . What remains invisible in researchers' assumptions, approaches, and conversations about non-white young people and health is the way the Anglo-American children's body size and shape are constructed as the norm, hierarchically superior to those of minorities, and the way dieting, fitness practices, and fat-phobic values are rooted historically in Anglo-American culture.
>
> (Azzarito 2009: 185–186)

Notice here what appears to be a claim to know what goes on in the minds (i.e. their 'assumptions') of obesity researchers and the conversations they have with each other. Whatever else we might say about them, obesity researchers regularly discuss the way particular technical cut-off points for overweight and obesity may be inappropriate for certain ethnic groups. Likewise, the question of developing forms of intervention that are culturally appropriate are also regularly debated in the literature. Some of us may not be unimpressed with the answers they arrive at, but it is simply untrue that these subtleties are 'invisible' to obesity researchers.

Echoing a general critique of science and medicine, in a series of publications Jutel (2001, 2005, 2006, 2009) has made the case that, from the late-nineteenth century onwards, general practice medicine became preoccupied with numerical measurement and visual inspection, at the same time turning away from the life narratives and subjective experiences of patients:

> I argue that an attraction to quantification and a belief that appearance mirrors the 'true' inner self, compounded by a religious fascination in establishing rules of normality, underpins a medical and cultural over-reliance on weight as an indicator of health. The lean, spare body is a 'good body,' evidence

of strong moral fiber, of someone who, constantly vigilant, 'looks after themselves.'

(2001: 283)

While Jutel's analysis does not stress the gendered dimensions of the medicalisation of fatness, her critique of both quantification and the centrality of the visual in obesity medicine rehearse the feminist critique of science in obvious ways. Likewise, her interest in the neo-liberal 'vigilant' self-governing subject is equally clear. Taken together, Jutel asks us to understand modern concerns about body weight via particular ways of doing science and medicine (impersonal, quantitative and normalising) and particular ways of being a modern neo-liberal citizen (self-governing and performative) . This is a very similar formulation to the one used by Monoghan (2007, 2008) in his discussions of men's body weight. Monoghan sees obesity science and its accompanying public health rhetoric as having promoted the 'McDonaldising' of men's bodies. In other words, obesity science, which Monoghan repeatedly accuses of being 'fat-phobic', has generated medical and commercial processes and rationalities preoccupied with the calculability, efficiency, predictability and control of human flesh.

Let me be clear. The authors cited here address a variety of concerns and research problems. What they share, though, is a conceptual language, landscape and trajectory. That is, their scepticism of obesity science is easily and quickly linked to wider concerns about neo-liberal morality, a morality that Halse (2009) calls 'virtue discourse'. Taken together, it is difficult to avoid the conclusion that these authors see obesity science and medicine as oppressive forces, more concerned with morality than health. In fact, Monoghan makes precisely this point: 'I would maintain that the institutionalised attack on fat is really about bodily regulation, morality and other sociological concerns (e.g. individualizing and de-politicizing healthism, the expansion of markets) rather than actually promoting biomedical health in the population' (2007: 70). This extraordinary claim is echoed, albeit with tongue apparently in cheek, by Halse:

> Because governments and their agents have committed intense political energy and considerable financial resources to constructing the bio-citizen, the virtue discourse of a normative BMI is not an innocent bystander in cho-reographing the future. But what has been buried in the jetsam and flotsam of its wake are bigger, more difficult issues: hunger; poverty; physical abuse; lack of fresh water, medical care and education; discrimination and inequali-ties; social and economic disadvantage. A cynic might wonder if this is a stratagem – a bio-political ruse – by governments and their agents to deflect the citizenry's attention from the social justice issues that continue to blight the lives of individuals and the well-being of communities and nations.
>
> (2009: 57)

Monaghan (2008) goes even further. Not only are obesity science and institutional medicine responsible for diverting attention away from what he sees as more pressing health concerns, they are also actually oppressing fat people. This is a view he makes clear with his use of the term 'militarised medicine' to describe the words and actions of researchers and clinical practitioners. Here, militarised medicine is a form of what he calls 'symbolic violence' that wreaks both psychological and physical harm.

Monaghan is particularly aggrieved at the militaristic metaphors that obesity science and medicine use. He offers this as evidence for either malicious intent or the cause of harmful side effects. And yet Monaghan seems unaware that science and medicine have used aggressive and militaristic metaphors for centuries, a point made for many years by feminist scholars (Reed 1976; Lloyd 1984; Easlea 1987). In fact, militaristic metaphors are used in almost every major area of social policy that come to my mind: the 'war drugs', the 'war on poverty' and many others. There is nothing new here. For better or worse, in recent decades obesity has found itself the subject of intense scientific and medical attention, a situation that was bound to precipitate the use of words like 'fighting' and 'war'. It is what science and medicine have always done when talking about the objects of their enquiry. This is neither the least bit remarkable, nor is drawing attention to it particularly enlightening.

There is a lurking confusion operating in the work of some obesity sceptics who try to use feminist theory and the critique of neo-liberalism to explain the obesity epidemic. It is perfectly reasonable to dispute the grounds upon which health authorities have chosen to embark on a war against fatness. Sceptics should and, in my view, must continue to dispute the exaggerated and plainly incorrect scientific claims made by obesity experts, health authorities and anyone else who speaks on the matter. Likewise, we must continue to point out the futility and potential harmful side effects of misguided anti-obesity policies. However, if health authorities arrive at a different view about the obesity epidemic from the one that sceptics would prefer and then go on to advocate for this view, this fact alone is not proof of a moral crusade or an attempt to divert attention away from more difficult health problems. Those who want to see the obesity epidemic as an example of neo-liberal thinking need to remember that the ranks of obesity experts are full of people campaigning to curb, tax and punish the behaviour of large corporations and who speak clearly and consistently about the futility of blaming individuals and focusing on personal responsibility. For some ideological sceptics, it seems that the only acceptable position for medical and public health authorities to take is to say nothing about obesity, which, of course, is not something they can do if we accept – and I think we have no choice but to accept – that most obesity experts honestly think that obesity is a serious health issue that needs to be fixed. In other words, the confusion here is between, on the one hand, a legitimate right of sceptics to probe and dispute the claims and practices of the advocates for a war on obesity and, on the other hand, a purely speculative and moralistic claim to know the motivations for this war better than the people who are prosecuting it. What is perhaps most dangerous is the way some ideological sceptics clearly assume that obesity scientists and clinicians are ignorant of the subtleties and risks involved in trying to reduce obesity at a population or individual level. Even a brief survey of the research literature shows that many obesity experts understand that their course of action is not risk free, but they have made the decision that there is greater risk in not doing anything. They are entitled to this view. The fact that they hold this view makes them, in my view, mistaken. It does not make them fat-haters or less intelligent or more right wing or more beguiled by the power of numbers or less concerned with the well-being of women or children or black people. Indeed, one of the most curious things about some obesity scepticism is how nasty, foolish and unprincipled it assumes people who work in mainstream obesity science and medicine to be.

Enemies and friends

A short digression before moving to the final sections of this chapter. In early 2008 I attended a small obesity-focused conference for general practice physicians. The core of the conference's program was a series of eight lectures, four of my own and four by the leading Canadian obesity researcher and clinician, Arya Sharma.

Sharma's position in the war on obesity is worth considering for a moment. While we differed greatly in our assessment of the medical implications of rising population body weights, there was much else in his four presentations that I think we might profitably juxtapose against Monaghan's idea of militarised medicine and Murray's disciplinary medicine. Sharma is the director of one of the largest obesity intervention facilities in the world, based in Edmonton, Canada. The facility performs a significant percentage of the bariatric surgery procedures that take place in Canada. Sharma argues that there should be more federal government support for the procedure. He argues this partly because demand for it hugely outstrips supply and because it is by far the best treatment available. He makes the point that (largely epidemiological) research into people's lifestyles has not delivered knowledge which is useful in helping very large people. In this context, no knowledge means no hope for people who want help.

Some readers may recall that the lack of useful knowledge generated by obesity research was one of the core points Jan Wright and I made in *The Obesity Epidemic* (Gard and Wright 2005). Overall, we also concurred with other obesity sceptics who have reserved particularly severe scorn for the advocates of bariatric surgery and the makers of weight loss drugs. Interestingly, though, Sharma's view was that surgery and drugs are the only two bright spots on the horizon for obesity treatment. Pointing out that it has never been difficult to achieve short-term weight loss, Sharma argues that surgery and weight loss drugs (and, often, a combination of the two) are the only proven methods for achieving long-term weight reduction.

In passing, I have regular contact with obesity sceptics, particularly those coming from a fat acceptance point of view, who take a particularly dim view of bariatric surgery. Putting to one side the fact that bariatric surgery takes the unhealthiness of obesity as a given, some argue that the procedures are dangerous and often have modest benefits. In other words, there is a tendency to see the matter in quite clear-cut, even moral terms. There are obvious grounds for taking this position, but there is surely another way of looking at the issue. As the historian of medicine

Roy Porter (2002) shows, many of the life-saving and health-improving surgeries that we take for granted today had extremely inauspicious beginnings. This was especially so in the twentieth century. Procedures such as organ transplantation initially claimed so many lives that its pioneers where excoriated for continuing to perform it and some simply stopped (see also Le Fanu 2000 on twentieth-century medicine and Ackerman 1999 for a bariatric surgeon's perspective). Can we be sure that bariatric surgery, as crude as it may currently seem, is the wrong thing to do, particularly given that we cannot just demand that everyone should be obesity sceptics?

Like other obesity researchers, Sharma also argues that rising obesity levels are a product of 'normal behaviour in an abnormal environment'; that is, people doing their best in difficult circumstances not of their own choosing. While some of us might have difficulty with the idea of normal and abnormal environments, the humanitarian impulse here is clear. Sharma argues that it is not acceptable to blame people for being obese; we have created a world in which it is more difficult not to be obese than in previous generations. In radically medicalising obesity, he argues that we need to think of obese people as ill and, therefore, deserving our support. Very few people advocate against making government-subsidised medical procedures available to people with smoking-related diseases or people injured by participating in high-risk activities like rock climbing or motor bike riding. Why then should we not extend the full reach of state medical care to obese people, particularly if obese people are over-represented amongst the poor?

In this admittedly isolated example, who is the friend of obese people? Professor Sharma or the obesity sceptics who argue, as I have, that we should not medicalise fatness and that we should not divert too much government money toward fighting obesity? It was also interesting to see that most, or perhaps all, of the forty or fifty family doctors present at the conference seemed sympathetic to the idea that we should not treat obese people as a body weight or BMI number in need of reduction, but rather as human beings with a complex range of potential medical needs. There was no obesity firing squad here.

Who killed medicine?

Finally, I want to consider two obesity sceptics who could easily have been included amongst Chapter 6's 'hard men'. In fact, both were contributors to the book *Panic Nation* and have pursued a generally libertarian line of argument in their numerous newspaper on online columns. I include them here, though, with a view to offering an alternative to some of the ideologically sceptical arguments we have encountered in this chapter.

In *The Rise and Fall of Modern Medicine*, James Le Fanu (2000) describes the period between the late 1930s and the mid-1970s as twentieth-century medicine's 'golden age'. It was a time in which huge advances in the treatment of a wide range of diseases were made by small groups of researchers working with rudimentary technology and without sophisticated knowledge of the biological processes in which their work intervened. Le Fanu characterises the period following the golden age as modern medicine's 'fall'. He does this for a number of reasons. In simple terms, the number of new cures began to decline rapidly at the same time as scientific understanding of human biology was improving dramatically. Le Fanu's argument is that, rather than improving things, technological advances have simply industrialised medicine while hugely adding to its costs. Although less thoroughly explored, Le Fanu's fall is also marked by the general population's embrace of 'alternative medicine' and the steady demoralisation of the medical profession.

However, the bulk of Le Fanu's analysis of modern medicine's decline centres on the emergence of 'the new genetics' and what he calls 'the social theory' of health. The genetic part of this analysis, concerned with what he sees as the over-selling of molecular biology as the new great medical frontier, is less relevant here. His discussion of the social theory, on the other hand, offers a telling counterpoint against the idea that medicine per se is the dupe of neo-liberal ideology, involved in a conspiracy, intended or not, against overweight and obese people.

Le Fanu's (2000) social theory is related to, but not the same thing as, what has become known as the 'new public health'. He locates the origins of the social theory in the pioneering work of Ansel Keys and Jeremiah Stamler in the 1950s and the emergence of the epidemiology of chronic 'lifestyle' diseases. The epidemiological turn moved the business of medicine away from the biological body – the site that had served it so well – towards lifestyle and the environment. For Le Fanu, this meant and continues to mean that the biological causes of so-called 'chronic diseases', like heart disease and diabetes, have gone relatively unexplored. The example of peptic ulcer is emblematic here, a condition that until the 1980s was generally assumed to be the product of bad diets, nervous personalities and stressful environments. The causal role of the helicobacter bacterium went undiscovered until 1984 when a novice Australian researcher saw through his microscope the bacterium that his more experienced colleagues had simply trained themselves not to see.

For Le Fanu, the social theory was, in essence, the virulent emergence of epidemiology as a force in medical research. He sees the increasing focus on lifestyle and environment from the 1960s onwards as a kind of virus invading the body of medicine. What is interesting here is that Le Fanu (2000) critiques the lifestyle-focused social theory in much the same way as empirical sceptics (see Chapter 6) have attacked obesity science. That is, Le Fanu is convinced that the social theory was based on flawed research but gained sway because its main protagonists infiltrated influential committees and powerful policy-making bodies; in short, bad ideas and self-interest. Taken from this angle, Le Fanu echoes the likes of Campos, Oliver and Monaghan: the war on lifestyle, like the war on obesity, is a kind of conspiracy. And yet there is a subtle but important distinction here. For some empirical and ideological sceptics, the conspiracy is perpetrated by medicine on the general public, while Le Fanu sees medicine and the people who practise and research it as the victims.

There is another crucial but easily overlooked difference between Le Fanu and the sceptics I have discussed above. As we saw, many sceptics argue that the obesity epidemic diverts attention away from the structural social determinants of health. For Le Fanu, however, the opposite is true: the increasing attention paid to lifestyle diseases, and eventually obesity, was caused by a preoccupation with a more holistic, structural, politically motivated view of health.

This point is vigorously taken up in Michael Fitzpatrick's (2001) *The Tyranny of Health*. Writing as a medical practitioner, Fitzpatrick argues that there has been far too much pressure placed on doctors to be their patients' lifestyle counsellors and less support for the day-to-day business of helping sick people to be well. While Le Fanu's (2000) perspective is historical, Fitzpatrick is concerned with the here-and-now fetishisation of health that values sheer longevity measured in years rather than quality of life. He complains that his consultation room is full of young and middle-aged 'worried well' who have been convinced by health authorities that death and disease lurk in every ache and pain.

Once again, the point here is that Fitzpatrick sees medicine itself as the casualty of an over-zealous public health policy environment. In considering the origins of these developments, Fitzpatrick concentrates on the rise of 'the new public health', a movement that from the 1970s sought to focus on the 'social determinants' of health. Many readers will be aware that 'the new public health' is a broad term, encompassing a variety of political agendas. However, I would offer that its central tenets stress:

- preventive medicine over curative medicine;
- epidemiological knowledge over anatomical/biological knowledge;
- holistic conceptions of health for groups of people over narrow conceptions of health for individuals;
- a generally liberal commitment to ameliorating health inequalities and supporting 'social justice'.

Both Le Fanu and Fitzpatrick see the new public health as well meaning but wrong headed and, most importantly, the primary source of contemporary panics about cholesterol, diet, obesity and the panoply of lifestyle diseases about which we are constantly reminded. The rhetoric of the new public health was hugely ambitious and assessed that, since epidemiology showed that health disparities correlated with differences on a number of social indices such as ethnicity, income and place of residence, huge improvements were yet possible. What was needed were interventions that altered the socially relevant factors that were amenable to manipulation. However, while many advocates of the new public health articulated something between frustration and hostility towards the power and hegemony of pathogen-focused scientific medicine, there was a demon lurking in their own vision; it was the demon of social control. After all, once you decide that people's social behaviours and context endanger their health, there is now only a short distance to coercive social policy.

Perhaps more important, both Le Fanu and Fitzpatrick argue that while the new public health sought to liberate people from modern, scientific, industrial medicine, it has had precisely the opposite effect. While the focus on lifestyle sought to give people the tools to take greater ownership of their own health, it has also given us weight loss pharmaceuticals, bariatric surgery, the 'healthy lifestyles' message and public health's war on obesity. While ideological sceptics blame neo-liberalism, Le Fanu and Fitzpatrick blame a mistaken preoccupation with social justice.

In some respects, these arguments are echoes of Crawford's (1980) classic paper 'Healthism and the medicalization of everyday life'. Like Le Fanu and Fitzpatrick, Crawford argues that despite apparently working in the opposite direction, the progressive health movements extended medical jurisdiction. He writes,

> If, in our enthusiasm for changes oriented toward creating new individual and social capacities freed from domination, we fail to identify aspects which may contradict those objectives, we risk repetitive disablement. Even the most radical challenges to orthodoxy are at best partial and always contain within their conceptions and structure the very elements against which the challenges are aimed. In the process, dominant ideologies and social structures are reproduced. Whether from external manipulation or internal conception (in some ways a false dichotomization), movements contain ideological contradictions from their inception.
>
> (1980: 367)

One aspect of Crawford's analysis is that by arguing that people could take greater control of their own health, we are now on the road to expecting that they should. Crawford was suspicious of the new public health movements because, despite loud assertions about radical change, they fostered:

> . . . a continued depoliticization and therefore undermining of the social effort to improve health and well-being. As an ideology which promotes heightened health awareness, along with personal control and change, it may prove beneficial for those who adopt a more health-promoting life style. But it may in the process also serve the illusion that we can *as individuals* control our existence, and that taking personal action to improve health will somehow satisfy the longing for a much more varied complex of needs.
>
> (1980: 368–369, emphasis in original)

In other words, it may not matter whether you see health as having primarily biological or social determinants or whether you see medicine as the hero or the villain; there is always a way to blame individuals for their health outcomes.

And yet, there is an important distinction to draw between Crawford, on the one hand, and Le Fanu and Fitzpatrick, on the other. While Crawford was at least in favour of the *spirit* of radical health politics, a politics that seeks to take health inequality seriously, Le Fanu and Fitzpatrick both see this as misguided. Fitzpatrick argues in some detail that huge improvements in the health of poorer Westerners have been achieved by virtue of steady economic development and free markets. Yes, differences in health outcomes for different social classes exist, but inequality is the price we must pay in capitalist systems for a general lifting of the base. While it is not my usual mode of argumentation to rejoice in capitalism's dividend to the poor, it is worth remembering that many obesity sceptics, including myself, have cited reports about the improving and generally unprecedented health outcomes achieved in modern Western countries. Fitzpatrick's argument is that these outcomes are one of the many dividends of liberal economic policies that reward innovation, investment and risk. In other words, people who decry structural inequalities must first show that structural inequality is a symptom of a failing system and not, in fact, a sign of success. Too often, Fitzpatrick argues, it is simply assumed that signs of inequality are proof of the need for radical change.

The poverty of moral critique

Where does all this leave us? In this and the previous chapter I have attempted to offer readers a sense of the diverse range of voices that have risen up against the idea of the obesity epidemic. It should surprise nobody that these voices speak from a wide and divergent cross-section of moral and ideological viewpoints. After all, obesity has become a complex and contentious social issue with the inevitable potential to both stimulate and irritate the sensibilities of just about anyone.

More important though, I have tried to offer an account of how different speakers appear to explain the obesity epidemic from their own narrowly partisan perspective. Not for a moment am I suggesting that this is a blindingly perceptive or original insight on my part. I am confident that most readers will have long ago understood the general point that we all think and speak from our own pre-existing preconceptions and moral framework. Certainly, in adding my own critical running commentary on obesity scepticism, I am not positioning myself as a neutral observer, although some readers will misunderstand this as my intention. With this accusation in mind, I ask readers to remember that the last two chapters were not written as mere surveys of a diverse literature. No doubt more contentiously, I have sought to go an extra step by trying to understand the shape of the arguments that sceptics make and, most important of all, how these arguments are made. It is a given, I think, that each of us is inclined to see our own explanations of phenomena as rational, coherent and based on an honest assessment of the evidence to hand. But this is surely never completely true for anyone. We all employ questionable assumptions as if they were cast-iron facts, and we all strategically and selectively include and exclude particular pieces of evidence. It is only through robust accounts of these complex and idiosyncratic manoeuvrings, even self-deceptions, that we can move to more intellectually sound and, I would add, ethically defensible positions. Critique is not the luxury of the researcher, scholar or intellectual; it is their responsibility.

As unremarkable as some might find my overall conclusions, nonetheless, I do think it is fascinating to register the sheer array of diametrically opposed interpretations within obesity scepticism. We have seen how some sceptics see the war on fatness as a concerted attack on capitalism, corporations and free markets and how others see it as an embodiment of corporatist, free-market, neo-liberal ways of thinking. There are those who blame mainstream science and others who lament the influence of mainstream science's enemies. Some use feminist theory as a weapon against obesity rhetoric, while others, in part, blame feminists for getting the whole thing started. In the hands of sceptics, the obesity epidemic is the product of both a naive preoccupation with, *and* an ignorance of, statistical data; both a politically motivated distraction from the structural causes of health inequality and the direct result of worrying too much about them. It is the isolated and recent work of a small but powerful clique of self-interested experts, but also symptomatic of the prejudices that have dogged the entirety of medical science for decades, if not centuries. It stems from thinking about health too biologically and not biologically enough, too socially and not socially enough. We have even encountered sceptics who blame the rise of obesity hysteria on a new puritanical aversion to pleasure and others who see it as a retreat from self-control and personal responsibility.

I will not go so far as to suggest that all these points of view are mistaken. I also fully accept that there is value in different interpretations of the same events and that it would be a terribly boring world if we slavishly restricted ourselves to beliefs with perfect internal coherence and external consistency. But I do think it is important to subject the work of sceptics to the same kind of scrutiny I have levelled at mainstream obesity rhetoric. Are all of these different sceptical interpretations equally valid? If not, what arguments and evidence would we muster in order to choose between them? Would we do more than simply retreat to our own particular theories and world views? In my opinion, nobody yet has adequately accounted for the rise of the obesity epidemic as an idea at a time of improving health around the Western world. This is not surprising; it is early days, the obesity epidemic's flame is only beginning to dim and the important histories of any event take time. This book is but a small contribution to this process.

For the moment, what has been most interesting to me is how few obesity sceptics are prepared to see themselves involved in a debate about obesity. With a few possible exceptions, sceptics tend to suspect obesity scientists and experts of some moral failing – misogyny, pecuniary self-interest, socialism, capitalism and a hatred of physical pleasure to name only a few. It is true that some of the critics of neo-liberalism argue that the obesity epidemic is not so much neo-liberal in its motivation but in its unintended effects. Still, we have seen how easy it is for this line of thinking to get personal; recall the way some critics of neo-liberalism assure us that the obesity epidemic is, in the end, a moral enterprise and essentially unconcerned with its purported goal of improving health. Gaesser, Campos and Oliver (see Chapter 6) are perhaps the most inclined to limit themselves to sorting out the truth about obesity as a health concern and, in a sense, to engage with obesity science on its own terms. While all three writers are happy to discuss the flow of money within obesity science and racial and gender prejudices, these issues are peripheral to their overall claim that overweight and obesity are not nearly the health risks we are constantly told they are.

Each of us is free to look for the deep, underlying causes of events, particularly globally significant events, that shape and impinge upon our lives. This is the role of scholars and intellectuals. But a serious danger lurks in this search: the more we try to delve into the psyches of our enemies, the more we end up simply discovering and describing ourselves. My social science colleagues call this the danger of constructing the 'other'. In our efforts to expose and demonise those with whom we disagree, we succeed only in creating a caricature that resembles nothing so much as our own fears, hopes and desires. This is precisely what happens when, as so many obesity sceptics do, we start from our pet theory or world view and then force obesity to look like all the other issues with which we have dealt in the past.

What is most tricky about the obesity epidemic, and what few sceptics seem prepared to admit, is that it is a broad social movement. It is not nor ever has been, as Campos and Oliver suggest, the province of a small group of east coast American health academics. The obesity epidemic is my family doctor, the coaches of the local junior sporting teams, journalists, politicians, academics from a bewildering array of sub-disciplines, aunts, uncles, friends and acquaintances. As some sceptics rightly point out, it has also been brewing for about 100 years. Explaining the obesity epidemic seems, at least to me, a similar kind of problem to explaining the 1960s or world wars, with all the potential for inaccuracy, exaggeration and partisan interpretation that these events invite.

To this end, most of the authors that I have discussed in this chapter have made important and thought-provoking contributions. Needless to say, many will also disagree vehemently with the assessment of this work that I have offered here. Once again, however, although it is something most readers will already appreciate, the point is still worth reiterating: whatever arguments we make about the origins or the consequences of the idea of an obesity epidemic, there is surely value in hesitating before presuming to know the minds of one's enemy better than they know it themselves.

8   The challenge of thinking well

I began writing this book in the latter half of 2008. There were signs even then that obesity was beginning to cool as a media story and public policy issue. In the previous five years or so it had competed successfully for attention with the likes of climate change and the risks of a new influenza pandemic. But as the decade drew to a close, various conflicts in the Middle East and the global economic downturn dominated the news. By the beginning of 2009, the obesity epidemic had become a second- or third-order problem for news and policy-makers.

The economic crisis of 2008 is perhaps not an unrelated ingredient here. Writing more than a decade ago, Stearns (1997) argued that while the twentieth century gave birth to a new and progressively more intense form of mass anti-fat sentiment, media and political concern about fatness has tended to wane during periods of economic downturn. In assessing the merits of this argument, it is worth pointing out that Stearns's central thesis is that anti-fat sentiment grew as other prejudices, such as those concerning social class, gender, race and sexual behaviour, became less socially acceptable. For Stearns, increasingly liberal and affluent Western societies have turned to fatness and thinness precisely because other markers have been drained of their ability to provoke prejudice and, therefore, confer status. This line of argument is similar to those who claim that Western affluence has generated anxiety about over-consumption, greed and a lack of restraint. Stearns' point is that anti-fat sentiment will resonate with people when affluence (and, therefore, anxiety about affluence) is greatest and decline when affluence declines. I am not aware of any other research to confirm this claim, and yet as I write in 2010 it feels like Stearns might have got it about right. With news that more than half a million Americans lost their job in December 2008 alone, the idea that the United States is a nation of fat over-consumers is likely to seem less credible. At the risk of trying to speak for others, my guess is that Stearns would say that we have moved into a period where the economic, cultural and social conditions are simply less conducive for generating worry about fatness.

Some readers might see this as a somewhat counter-intuitive conclusion. Surely greater economic hardship should make us more, not less, suspicious of over-consumption? And yet this would be to miss what, in the era of the obesity epidemic, was a subtle but crucial distinction between over-consumption, on the one hand, and lack of restraint, on the other. Obesity epidemic rhetoric told us that *everyone*, rich and poor, was getting fatter. It was for this reason that sceptics of obesity epidemic thinking have generally complained about a lack of concern for poorer people who live in environments more likely to make them fat. The insight that I take from all of this is that in the context of obesity epidemic rhetoric, over-consumption was less of a sin than a lack of restraint. As overweight and obesity statistics repeatedly showed, the biggest consumers in Western societies (wealthier people) were not the fattest. High levels of consumption could be forgiven so long as consumers could demonstrate a modicum of restraint, a task for which having a slim body is perfectly suited.

Still, there is an obvious problem with this line of argument, a problem that has been particularly evident in much of the more social science-minded scepticism I discussed in Chapter 7. Many sceptics are determined to argue that contemporary obesity anxiety is the result of deep-seated cultural anxieties and prejudices, be they against fat people or women or the poor or ethnic minorities. Like Stearns, other sceptics look to history and find earlier examples of when the pressure to be thin increased. Armed with these examples, they conclude that today's obesity epidemic is either an echo of past anxieties and prejudices or perhaps a more virulent outbreak of a cultural disease that lies dormant before periodically flaring into life.

What this analysis overlooks is that the twenty-first century's obesity epidemic was, to a large degree, fuelled by statistics. In their rush to accuse obesity science of fat hatred and prejudice, many sceptics sidestepped overweight and obesity statistics and, therefore, in one gloriously misguided manoeuvre rendered themselves irrelevant, disqualifying themselves from contributing to discussion about what was going on now.

Some readers will now sniff a contradiction in my argument. If the obesity epidemic is a complex social movement, as I have just claimed, surely the thing to do is to look for the underlying social and cultural currents that created the conditions for this movement to take place? Surely these currents are precisely the kinds of anxieties and prejudices to which the ideological sceptics have drawn attention? The problem here is that in falling back on standard political tropes like class, gender and race, many sceptics have not recognised the ways in which today's obesity epidemic is its own unique social phenomenon. In fact, if I have succeeded in convincing readers about nothing else in this book, I would settle for having at least clarified the way all commentators, alarmists and sceptics tend to speak from narrow personal perspectives. While alarmists tend to myopically assert that obesity is amongst the greatest threats to human kind, sceptics tend to completely ignore the work of obesity scientists, tossing it aside with a moral slur or the flick of a generalisation or two.

I do not say that people should never speak from their own point of view or that no good can ever come from it when they do. And yet from my own (no doubt narrow) perspective, it is curious that the apparent empirical reality of increasing fatness is hardly ever mentioned by sceptics. Why is it so difficult to factor this into a sophisticated social science account of the obesity epidemic without falling into naive scientism? I submit that many obesity sceptics, particularly those I have categorised as 'ideological', have avoided talking about obesity statistics because they simply have not known what to say about them. This is perhaps reasonable when preaching to the converted but not if our mission is to change minds or explain a complex epidemiological phenomenon.

Moreover, so little critical obesity research has actually attempted to understand the ways in which Western food cultures have changed how people eat or the way modern media cultures are re-shaping desires and appetites. Physical exercise, too, has been turned into a commodity – in some cases, a very expensive commodity. Isn't this significant? Like most sceptics, I think we need to do much better than the crude and simplistic explanations offered by obesity science. But what, at present, are our alternatives? The wholly unsatisfactory genetic arguments of fat acceptance? The pleas from social science that we not blame individuals? The conspiracy theories of the neo-liberals and industry lobbyists? Once again, I think the work of authors like Campos and Oliver have so far come closest to treating the obesity epidemic as a unique social phenomenon that is both connected but also irreducible to others. But even here we are only at the beginning, not the destination. Oliver, for example, says that the most significant change to the way Westerners eat is increased between-meal snacking. Is this credible? Is this really the only significant change to Western food cultures playing a role in rising body weights? The proportionally small but interesting spike in the number of extremely obese people is, I think, telling us something about the food cultures we are creating. Something more than a little extra between meal snacking is surely going on. Obesity scientists can see plainly that the world has changed and they simply cannot understand why obesity sceptics seem not to want to acknowledge this.

As I have said, I think the obesity epidemic is best thought of as a complex social movement and not, as obesity alarmists argue, the simple sum total of small changes in the way we eat and move our bodies. It has taken place in public health authority offices, school classrooms, supermarkets, on television and in the minds of average citizens. As Chapter 5 of this book tried to show, it is also having a wide range of consequences that have little to do with reducing body weight. In fact, like all globally pervasive shifts in the way people think and behave, perhaps a comprehensive understanding of what the obesity epidemic is and how it happened is beyond any of us and a smorgasbord of interpretations is the best we can hope for. Still, in trying to manage this complexity, some obesity sceptics have sought the safe waters of moral certainty, offering that their version of events is not only more trustworthy, but also more noble and ethical than mainstream obesity science. I have to say that in attempting to bring arguments against the idea of an obesity epidemic I have wrestled over whether my scholarship does society a service or a disservice. When other sceptics describe the obesity epidemic as a 'myth' or a 'lie' or a form of 'oppression' or 'symbolic violence' they announce that they, the sceptics, have the interests of society at heart and that their opponents do not. I am afraid I lack this moral conviction. I have satisfied myself that the role of the sceptical scholar is a modest one, offering people alternative ways of thinking rather than trying to arbitrate the moral worth of different points of view.

It seems beyond doubt that Western obesity rates increased in the twenty or thirty years prior to 2000. At this moment my view is that many of those who study obesity and work with obese people allowed themselves to be spooked and hit the panic button. For reasons best known only to themselves, they assumed that the increases they saw would go on unchanged into the future. Some made the mistake of assuming that because rates of increase had changed, rates of increase would go on changing. This perhaps explains how the word 'exponential' crept into obesity discourse.

I have no reason to doubt the many researchers, clinicians and health experts with whom I have spoken over the last ten years who say they are seeing more overweight and obese people. I do not see any point denying that increased body weight will result in some level of strain on Western and, in the future, non-Western medical systems. I also find it difficult to imagine that Western life expectancies will go on increasing for ever and I do no think that all the social changes wrought by global capitalism are likely to result in better health.

However, I do believe that genetics tells us nothing very interesting at all about weight change at the individual or population level. I believe that Western populations have grown slightly fatter over the last thirty years. I believe that this change must be the result of less exercise and greater caloric intake – not genetics – but that the relative contribution of either has varied from context to context and will never be known in any simple, global sense. There will never be a scientific answer for why the obesity epidemic happened.

I am also inclined to wonder whether the idea of an obesity epidemic appeared as an oasis of simplicity in the face of more troubling complexities. Was it a much-needed distraction from the immense contradictions and anxieties produced by having better general health as well as hugely and perhaps unsustainably expensive modern health systems? It is surely curious that at a time when the costs of keeping people alive longer and longer are becoming ever more apparent, we are swamped by the idea that our health systems will collapse under the weight of people dying young. For example, the United Kingdom's Change4Life anti-obesity public health campaign exists apparently to stave off a costly epidemic of early British deaths, a situation that, if it ever actually happened, would in purely economic terms result in considerable health cost savings.

The question raised in the first few chapters of this book, though, is whether the obesity epidemic amounts to a health crisis. During the final days of writing this book a number of scientists called global warming the greatest threat to humanity. Is obesity really in this league of problems as some obesity experts claimed? I think we can now call the bluff of obesity science. The studies pointing to the ambiguous relationship between body weight, health and mortality are piling up. Of course it is not healthy to be extremely fat, but the most important reason why there never was, nor will be, an obesity health crisis in the foreseeable future is because overweight and moderate obesity, in and of themselves, are neither diseases nor particularly bad for one's health.

There is much about this book that is speculative. I have no crystal ball and it is possible, of course, that overweight and obesity prevalence will soon start rapidly increasing around the Western world despite the recent lulls that I described in Chapter 3. Still, I think this is unlikely. A famous Australian state premier once joined a group of end-of-the-world Christians on an Adelaide beach to demonstrate that he did not believe the catastrophic tidal wave that they predicted was coming. Yes, body weight will be a feature of our public health landscape for a long time to come, but there will be no obesity tidal wave. In fact, obesity is a very small challenge compared with the formidable and looming financial sustainability pressures that await Western health systems; pressures that are systemic in nature and have little do with any particular disease or family of diseases.

To conclude then, I want to emphasise that this has been a book about an idea, not about people. Where did this idea come from? How did it spread? How have people responded to it? When did it begin to die? When I have talked about the end of the obesity epidemic I have tried to limit myself to evidence of its death as an idea. This is why I think overweight and obesity statistics are crucial: they have been central to obesity rhetoric over the last ten years in a way that, to my knowledge, they have not been during earlier spikes in body weight anxiety. As the flattening of overweight and obesity statistics becomes more widely known, I expect the obesity epidemic's proponents to ratchet up the intensity of their rhetoric once more because they will sense a shift in the rhetorical climate against them. However, they will find to their surprise that the rhetorical landscape has shifted. The voices of scepticism are now more numerous and well organised. Sceptical online blogs and discussion groups are multiplying – evidence, I think, that the obesity epidemic has generated its own popular backlash and that one need not be an epidemiologist or social theorist to perceive the mistakes and exaggerations of obesity science. It would be ludicrous to say that because there are voices calling for the end of racism that, therefore, racism has ended, just as simply saying that global warming is a myth does not make it so. However, the voices of obesity scepticism are now moving into the mainstream and there is a credible scientific, medical and historical story for us to tell.

In an attempt to deflect some of the arguments I have raised in this book, a few obesity scientists have suggested to me that, since many researchers can now see that obesity has peaked and may be on the way down, the challenge ahead will be to convince politicians who have become true believers in the war on fatness. This is a self-serving and mistaken view. By and large, I think most politicians would welcome the news that the obesity epidemic is over, breath a sigh of relief and move on to the next problem. Neither politicians nor journalists created the obesity epidemic and compared it to plague, global warming or terrorism. The challenge for the future will be to change the minds of the scientists – nobody else – and to shape the anti-obesity policy landscape, the legacy of the last ten years, so that it is more humane, less wasteful and more likely to have spinoff benefits. Debates about the causes of the obesity epidemic are now essentially over and the next decade will be more about mending and managing the fall-out of the previous decades' rhetorical excesses.

References

Ackerman, N. B. (1999) *Fat No More: The Answer for the Dangerously Overweight*, New York: Prometheus Books.

Ackerman, T. (2002) 'Study shows Houston kids getting fatter', *The Houston Chronicle*, 23 January: A-19.

Adams, M. (2004) 'Obesity epidemic threatens to bankrupt U.S. economy and threaten financial stability of the world', *NaturalNews.com*. Online. Available at: http://www.naturalnews.com/001516.html (accessed 15 March 2009).

Adler, N. E. and Stewart, J. (2009) 'Reducing obesity: motivating action while not blaming the victim', *The Milbank Quarterly* 87, 1: 49–70.

Aeberli, I., Ammann, R. S., Knabenhans, M., Molinari, L. and Zimmermann, M. B. (2009) 'Decrease in the prevalence of paediatric adiposity in Switzerland from 2002 to 2007', *Public Health Nutrition*: doi:10.1017/S1368980009991558.

Aichroth, M. (2005) 'Sports and exercise', in S. Feldman and V. Marks (eds) *Panic Nation: Unpicking The Myths We're Told About Food And Health*, London: John Blake: 261–268.

Alabama State Employees Insurance Board. (n.d.) *State of Alabama Wellness Premium Discount Program*. Online. Available at: http://www.alseib.org/PDF/SEHIP/SEHIPWellnessPremiumDiscount.pdf (accessed 18 March 2010).

Albemarle State Policy Center. (2008) '2007 End of year report: A report on state action to promote nutrition, increase physical activity and prevent obesity', *Balance*, 5. Online. Available at: http://www.rwjf.org/childhoodobesity/product.jsp?id=31471 (accessed 18 March 2010).

Albemarle State Policy Center. (2009) 'Fall 2008 report: A report on state action to promote nutrition, increase physical activity and prevent obesity', *Balance*, 7. Online. Available at: http://www.rwjf.org/files/research/30792.balancefall2008.pdf (accessed 18 March 2010).

Alexander, M. (2008) 'How to tackle the obesity explosion', *Western Daily Press*, 12 September.

Allison, D. B., Fontaine, K. R., Manson, J. E., Stevens, J. and VanItallie, T. (1999) 'Annual deaths attributable to obesity in the United States', *Journal of the American Medical Association* 282, 16: 1530–1538.

American Health Network. (2005) 'EU food industry called to battle against obesity'. Online. Available at: http://www.health.am/weightloss/more/eu_food_industry_called_to_battle_against_obesity/ (accessed 11 December 2009).

American Obesity Association. (2005) 'American Obesity Association hails Medicare decision'. Online. Available at: http://obesity1.tempdomainname.com/subs/pressroom/medicare2004.shtml (accessed 12 August 2008).

Amler, R. W. and Eddins, D. L. (1987) 'Cross-sectional analysis: precursors of premature death in the United States', *American Journal of Preventive Medicine* 3(suppl):
181–187.

Anderssen, S. A., Engeland, A., Søgaard, A. J., Nystad, W., Graff-Iversen, S. and Holme, I.
(2008) 'Changes in physical activity behavior and the development of body mass index
during the last 30 years in Norway', *Scandinavian Journal of Medicine and Science in
Sports* 18, 3: 309–317.

Arkansas Department of Education (2005) 'Nutrition standards and allowable foods/
beverages with maximum portion size restrictions', *Arkansas Department of Education,
Commissioner's Communication*. Online. Available at: http://cnn.k12.ar.us/Topics%
20of%20Interest/Program%20Operations/Directors%20Memos/2006%20Memos/
FIN-06-016.htm (accessed 18 March 2010).

Australian Institute of Health and Welfare. (2008) *Australia's health 2008*, Cat. no. AUS
99, Canberra: AIHW.

Australian Science Media Centre. (2009) 'New obesity figures from the National Survey of
Health – experts react'. Online. Available at: http://www.aussmc.org/National_Health_
Survey.php (accessed 14 January 2009).

Azzarito, L. (2009) 'The rise of the corporate curriculum: fatness, fitness, and whiteness',
in J. Wright and V. Harwood (eds) *Biopolitics and the 'Obesity Epidemic': Governing
Bodies*, New York: Routledge: 183–196.

Barnett, G. (2006) 'Obesity starts in the home – treating it can start in the doctor's surgery'. Online. Available at: http://www.guybarnett.com/index.php?page=show_
article&artid=586 (accessed 28 September 2006).

Basham, P., Gori, G. and Luik, J. (2006) *Diet Nation: Exposing the Obesity Crusade*,
London: The Social Affairs Unit.

Baum, C. (2007) 'The effects of race, ethnicity, and age on obesity', *Journal of Population
Economics* 20, 3: 687–705.

Bennett, K., Kabir, Z., Unal, B., Shelley, E., Critchley, J., Perry, I., Feely, J. and Capewell,
S. (2006) 'Explaining the recent decrease in coronary heart disease mortality rates
in Ireland, 1985–2000', *Journal of Epidemiology and Community Health* 60, 4:
322–327.

Berentzen, T. and Sørensen, T. I. A. (2007) 'Physical inactivity, obesity and health',
Scandinavian Journal of Medicine and Science in Sports 17, 4: 301–302.

Blackburn, G. L. and Waltman, B. A. (2005) 'Expanding the limits of treatment – new
strategic initiatives', *Journal of The American Dietetic Association* 105, 5(suppl. 1):
S131–S135.

Bleich, S., Cutler, D., Murray, C. and Adams, A. (2008) 'Why is the developed world
obese?', *Annual Review of Public Health* 29: 273–295.

BNET. (2008) 'Obesity epidemic seen slowing but not falling'. Online. Available at: http://
findarticles.com/p/articles/mi_m3374/is_13_30/ai_n30977455/ (accessed 10 April
2010).

Bonfiglioli, C., King, L., Smith, B., Chapman, S. and Holding, S. (2007) 'Obesity in the
media: political hot potato or human interest story?', *Australian Journalism Review* 29,
1: 53–61.

Booth, M. L., Chey, T., Wake, M., Norton, K., Hesketh, K., Dollman, J. and Robertson, I.
(2003) 'Change in the prevalence of overweight and obesity among young Australians,
1969–1997', *American Journal of Clinical Nutrition* 77, 1: 29–36.

Bray, G. A. and Popkin, B. M. (1998) 'Dietary fat intake does affect obesity!', *American
Journal of Clinical Nutrition* 68, 6: 1157–1173.

Breen, H. B. and Ireton-Jones, C. S. (2004) 'Predicting energy needs in obese patients', *Nutrition in Clinical Practice* 19, 3: 284–289.

Brignell, J. (2000) *Sorry, Wrong Number! The Abuse of Measurement*. Great Britain: Brignell Associates.

British Heart Foundation. (2009) 'Prevalence of obesity, adults aged 16-64, 1986/87-2004, England'. Online. Available at: http://www.heartstats.org/atozpage.asp?id=1364 (accessed 15 December 2009).

Brownell, K. D. and Horgen, K. B. (2004) *Food Fight: The Inside Story of the Food Industry, America's Obesity Crisis, and What We Can Do About It*, Chicago: Contemporary Books.

Brownell, K. D. and Warner, K. E. (2009) 'The perils of ignoring history: Big Tobacco played dirty and millions died. How similar is Big Food?', *The Milbank Quarterly* 87, 1: 259–294.

Budd, G. M. and Hayman, L. L. (2008) 'Addressing the childhood obesity crisis: a call to action', *American Journal of Maternal Child Nursing* 33, 2: 111–118.

Bunting, C. (2002) 'Healthy diet? Eat your words', *The Times Higher*, 15 April: 16–17.

Burdette, H. L. and Whitaker, R. C. (2004) 'Neighborhood playgrounds, fast food restaurants, and crime: relationships to overweight in low-income preschool children', *Preventive Medicine* 38, 1: 57–63.

Burkhauser, R. V., Cawley, J. and Schmeiser, M. D. (2009) 'The timing of the rise in U.S. obesity varies with measures of fatness', *Economics and Human Biology* 7, 3: 307–318.

Burrows, L. (2004) 'Understanding and investigating cultural perspectives in physical education', in J. Wright, D. Macdonald and L. Burrows (eds) *Critical Inquiry and Problem-Solving in Physical Education*, London: Routledge: 105–119.

Burrows, L. (2009) 'Pedagogizing families through obesity discourse', in J. Wright and V. Harwood (eds) *Biopolitics and the 'Obesity Epidemic': Governing Bodies*, New York: Routledge: 127–140.

Burros, M. and Warner, M. (2006) 'Bottlers agree to a school ban on sweet drinks', *The New York Times*. Online. Available at: http://www.nytimes.com/2006/05/04/health/04soda.html?_r=1 (accessed 18 March 2010).

Byrd, S. (2009) 'Health message strong in Mississippi schools', Associated Press State and Local Wire, 9 October.

Caballero, B. (2007) 'The global epidemic of obesity: an overview', *Epidemiologic Reviews* 29, 1: 1–5.

Caballero, B., Clay, T., Davis, S. M., Ethelbah, B., Rock, B. H., Lohman, T., Norman, J., Story, M., Stone, E. J., Stephenson, L., Stevens, J. and Pathways Study Research Group (2003) 'Pathways: a school-based, randomized controlled trial for the prevention of obesity in American Indian schoolchildren', *American Journal of Clinical Nutrition* 78, 5: 1030–1038.

California Association for Physical Education, Recreation and Dance. (2009) 'Physical education and marching band, JROTC and other Single Activities'. Online. Available at: http://www.cahperd.org/legislation/images/PE-Marching%20Band%20JROTC.pdf (accessed 10 April 2010).

California Department of Education. (2009) *Program Overview: Overview of the California Fitness Test Program*. Online. Available at: http://www.cde.ca.gov/ta/tg/pf/pftprogram.asp (accessed 24 March 2010).

California Department of Education, Communications Division. (2009) 'State schools chief Jack O'Connell teams up with Governor's Fitness Council chair Jake Steinfeld to release 2009 physical fitness results'. Online. Available at: http://www.cde.ca.gov/nr/ne/ yr09/yr09rel159.asp (accessed 24 March 2010).

Calloway, L. (2006) 'The war on Fluffernutter escalates in Legislature', *The Boston Globe*. Online. Available at: http://www.boston.com/news/local/articles/2006/06/21/the_war_ on_fluffernutter_escalates_in_legislature/ (accessed 18 March 2010).

Campos, P. (2004a) *The Obesity Myth: Why America's Obsession with Weight is Hazardous to your Health*, New York: Gotham Books.

Campos, P. (2004b) 'Why our fears about fat are misplaced', *New Scientist* 182, 2445: 20.

Campos, P., Saguy, A., Ernsberger, P., Oliver, E. and Gaesser, G. (2006) 'The epidemiology of overweight and obesity: public health crisis or moral panic', *International Journal of Epidemiology* 35, 1: 55–60.

Carvel, J. (2006) 'Child obesity has doubled in a decade', *The Guardian*, 22 April: 1–2.

CBS News. (2006) 'Obesity an "international scourge"'. Online. Available at: http://www. cbsnews.com/stories/2006/09/03/health/main1962961.shtml (accessed 26 June 2007).

Centers for Disease Control and Prevention. (2008) 'CDC Congressional Testimony'. Online. Available at: http://www.cdc.gov/washington/testimony/2008/t20080923.htm (accessed 10 December 2009).

Central Stickney School District #110. (2009) *Nutrition and Physical Activity Wellness Policy*. Online. Available at: http://www.sahs.k12.il.us/documents/WELLNESS%20POLICY. doc (accessed 18 March 2010).

Center for Consumer Freedom. (2005) *An Epidemic of Obesity Myths*, Washington, D.C.: The Center for Consumer Freedom.

Chakravarthy, M. V. and Booth, F. W. (2003) 'Inactivity and inaction: we can't afford either', *Archives of Pediatrics and Adolescent Medicine*, 157, 8: 731–732.

Chrisler, J. C. (1989) 'Should feminist therapists do weight loss counseling?', in L. S. Brown and E. D. Rothblum (eds) *Fat Oppression and Psychotherapy: A Feminist Perspective*, New York: The Haworth Press: 31–37.

Clinton Foundation. (2005) 'Creating a Healthier Generation'. Online. Available at: http:// www.clintonfoundation.org/050305-feature-wjc-aha-healthier-generation-initiative.htm (accessed 14 April 2008).

Clifton, J. (2010) 'Tipping the scales', *New Zealand Listener*, 23–29 January: 24–27.

Cole, M. (2009) 'Teachers want junk snacks back – for themselves', *The Oregonian*. Online. Available at: http://www.oregonlive.com/politics/oregonian/index.ssf?/base/ news/1234587316281120.xml&coll=7 (accessed 18 March 2010).

Council of State Governments. (2007) *Obesity Tool Kit*. Online. Available at: http://www. healthystates.csg.org/NR/rdonlyres/36F21685-38E8-44BC-9C06-1458515BE93E/0/ RWJtoolkitwhole.pdf (accessed 18 March 2010).

Cowley, G. (2000) 'Generation XXL', *Newsweek*, 3 July: 40–44.

Crawford, R. (1980) 'Healthism and the medicalization of everyday life', *International Journal of Health Services* 10, 3: 365–388.

CTV News. (2008) 'B.C. has lowest obesity levels in 10 years'. Online. Available at: http:// www.ctv.ca/servlet/ArticleNews/story/CTVNews/20080929/obesity_levels_080929/20 080929?hub=Canada (accessed 10 December 2009).

Czernichow, S., Vergnaud, A., Maillard-Teyssier, L., Péneau, S., Bertrais, S., Méjean, C., Vol, S., Tichet, J. and Hercberga, S. (2009) 'Trends in the prevalence of obesity in employed adults in central-western France: a population-based study, 1995–2005', *Preventive Medicine* 48, 3: 262–266.

Delpeuch, F., Maire, B., Monnier, E. and Holdsworth, M. (2009) *Globesity: A Planet Out of Control?*, London: Earthscan.

Department of Health. (2006) *Health Profile of England*, London: Department of Health.

Department of Human Services. (2008) *Future prevalence of overweight and obesity in Australian children and adolescents, 2005–2025*, Melbourne: Public Health Branch.

Devlin, K. (2008) 'Obesity rates "have hit their peak", conference to be told', *Telegraph Online*. Online. Available at: http://www.telegraph.co.uk/health/article3413490.ece (accessed 28 November 2008).

de Wilde, J. A., van Dommelen, P., Middelkoop, B. J. C. and Verkerk, P. H. (2009) 'Trends in overweight and obesity prevalence in Dutch, Turkish, Moroccan and Surinamese South Asian children in the Netherlands', *Archives of Disease in Childhood* 94, 10: 795–800.

DiabetesAnswers.org. (2004) 'Obesity epidemic threatens to bankrupt U.S. economy and threaten financial stability of the world'. Online. Available at: http://www.diabetesanswers. org/1444_health_obesity.html (accessed 15 March 2009).

Divine, M. (2004) 'Dying for another snack', *The Sun-Herald*, 30 May: 15.

Drake, J. (2002) 'Band leaders, PE advocates clash', *The State.com*. Online Available at: http://www.colorguardfloors.com/guardzone/PDF/PE_Credits_for_Band.pdf (accessed 15 March 2008)

Duval County Public Schools. (n.d.) *Wellness Program*. Online. Available at: http://www. duvalschools.org/static/students/lunch/DCPS%20Wellness%20Policy.pdf (accessed 18 March 2010).

Dyson, B., Amis, J., Wright, P., Vardaman, J. and Ferry, H. (forthcoming) 'The production, communication, and contestation of physical education policy: The cases of Mississippi and Tennessee', *Policy Futures in Education*.

Easlea, B. (1987) 'Patriarchy, scientists and nuclear warriors', in M. Kaufman *Beyond Patriarchy: Essays by Men on Pleasure, Power, and Change*, Toronto: Oxford University Press: 195–215.

Egger, G. J., Vogels, N. and Westerterp, K. R. (2001) 'Estimating historical changes in physical activity levels', *Medical Journal of Australia* 175, 11–12: 635–636.

English, S. (2005) 'The fattest children in the world', *Times Online*. Online. Available at: http://www.timesonline.co.uk/article/0,,8126-1922831,00.html (accessed 1 March 2006).

Enid Public Schools. (n.d.) *Wellness Guidelines*. Online. Available at: http://www. enidpublicschools.org/admin/health/wellness.pdf (accessed 18 March 2010).

Ernsberger, P. and Haskew, P. (1987) *Rethinking Obesity: An Alternative View of its Health Implications*, New York: Human Sciences Press.

Esmail, N. and Brown, J. (2005) 'The wrong defense for tackling obesity', *The Fraser Institute*. Online. Available at: http://www.fraserinstitute.ca/shared/readmore1. asp?sNav=ed&id=352 (accessed 3 November 2005).

EurekAlert. (2009) 'Increased food intake alone explains the increase in body weight in the United States'. Online. Available at: http://www.eurekalert.org/pub_releases/2009-05/eaft-ifi050709.php (accessed 17 May 2009)

Evans, B. (2006) '"Gluttony or sloth": critical geographies of bodies and morality in (anti)obesity policy', *Area* 38, 3: 259–267.

Evans, J. (2003) Physical education and health: a polemic or 'let them eat cake!', *European Physical Education Review*, 9(1): 87–101.

Evans, J., Rich, E., Davies, B. and Allwood, R. (2005) 'The embodiment of learning: what the sociology of education doesnít say about "risk" in going to school', *International Studies in Sociology of Education* 15, 2: 129–148.

Fallon, P., Katsman, M. A. and Wooley, S. C. (eds) (1994) *Feminist Perspectives on Eating Disorders*, New York: The Guilford Press.

Farrell, S. W., Braun, L., Barlow, C. E., Cheng, Y. J. and Blair, S. N. (2002) 'The relation of body mass index, cardiorespiratory fitness, and all-cause mortality in women', *Obesity Research*, 10, 6: 417–423.

Feldman, S. (2005) 'Junk food', in S. Feldman and V. Marks (eds) *Panic Nation: Unpicking The Myths We're Told About Food And Health*, London: John Blake: 61–65.

Feldman, S. and Marks, V. (eds) (2005) *Panic Nation: Unpicking The Myths We're Told About Food And Health*, London: John Blake.

Finkelstein, E. A. and Zuckerman, L. (2008) *The Fattening of America: How the Economy Makes US Fat, If It Matters, and What to Do About It*, Hoboken, New Jersey: John Wiley and Sons.

Fitzpatrick, M. (2001). *The Tyranny of Health: Doctors and the Regulation of Lifestyle*, London: Routledge.

Fitzpatrick, M. (2006) 'Stop bullying fat kids', *Spiked Online*. Online. Available at: http://www.spiked-online.com/index.php?/site/printable/315/ (accessed 28 November 2008).

Flegal, K. M., Carroll, M. D., Ogden, C. L. and Curtin, L. R. (2010) 'Prevalence and trends in obesity among US adults, 1999–2008', *Journal of the American Medical Association* 303, 3: 235–241.

Flegal, K. M., Graubard, B. I., Williamson, D. F. and Gail, M. H. (2005) 'Excess deaths associated with underweight, overweight and obesity', *Journal of the American Medical Association* 293, 15: 1861–1867.

Food Online. (2000) 'JAMA study documents 6% rise in obesity in US'. Online. Available at: http://www.foodonline.com/article.mvc/JAMA-study-documents-6-rise-in-obesity-in-US-0001?VNETCOOKIE=NO (accessed 24 April 2008).

Ford, E. S., Ajani, U. A., Croft, J. B., Critchley, J. A., Labarthe, D. R., Kottke, T. E., Giles, W. H. and Capewell S. (2007) 'Explaining the decrease in U.S. deaths from coronary disease, 1980-2000', *New England Journal of Medicine* 356, 23: 2388–2398.

Foresight. (2005) 'Tackling Obesities: Future Choice Projects'. Online. Available at: http://www.foresight.gov.uk/Obesity/Obesity.htm (accessed 14 December 2007).

Foreyt, J. P. (1997) 'An etiologic approach to obesity', *Hospital Practice* 32, 8: 123–124, 126, 128.

Fox, S. (2003) 'Children weighing more than 140 kg treated at hospital', *Fairfax New Zealand Limited*. Online. Available at: http://www.stuff.co.nz/stuff/0,2106,2746069a7144,00.html (accessed 3 December 2004).

Frank, A. (1993) 'Futility and avoidance: medical professionals in the treatment of obesity', *Journal of the American Medical Association* 269, 16: 2132–2133.

Frank, L. D., Andresen, M. A. and Schmid, T. L. (2004) 'Obesity relationships with community design, physical activity, and time spent in cars', *American Journal of Preventive Medicine* 27, 2: 87–96.

Frank, L. D., Engelke, P. O. and Schmid, T. L. (2003) *Health and Community Design: The Impact of the Built Environment on Physical Activity*, Washington, D.C.: Island Press.

French, S. A., Story, M. and Jeffery, R. W. (2001) 'Environmental influences on eating and physical activity', *Annual Review of Public Health* 22: 309–335.

Fullagar, S. (2003) 'Governing women's active leisure: the gendered effects of calculative rationalities within Australian health policy', *Critical Public Health* 13, 1: 47–60.

Fullagar, S. (2009) Governing healthy family lifestyles through discourses of risk and responsibility' in J. Wright and V. Harwood (eds) *Biopolitics and the 'Obesity Epidemic': Governing Bodies*, New York: Routledge: 108–126.

Gaesser, G. A. (2002) *Big Fat Lies: The Truth About Your Weight and Your Health*, Carlsbad: Gurze Books.

Gard, M. (2008) 'Producing little decision makers and goal setters in the age of the obesity crisis', *Quest* 60, 4: 488–502.

Gard, M. and Wright, J. (2005) *The Obesity Epidemic: Science, Morality and Ideology*, London: Routledge.

Garrison, T. N. and Levitsky, D. (1993) *Fed Up! A Woman's Guide to Freedom from the Diet/Weight Prison*, New York: Carroll and Graf Publishers.

Gibbs, W. W. (2005) 'Obesity: an overblown epidemic?', *Scientific American* 292, 6: 70.

Goldstein, H. (2009) 'Translating research into public policy', *Journal of Public Health Policy* 30(S1): S16–S20.

Goodman, K. K. (1989) 'Metamorphosis', in L. S. Brown and E. D. Rothblum (eds) *Fat Oppression and Psychotherapy: A Feminist Perspective*, New York: The Haworth Press: 11–18.

Grant, B. C. and Bassin, S. (2007) 'The challenge of paediatric obesity: more rhetoric than action', *New Zealand Medical Journal* 120, 1260: u2684.

Gray, V. and Holman, C. D. J. (2009) *Deaths and premature loss of life caused by over-weight and obesity in Australia in 2011–2050: Benefits from different intervention strategies*. Report for the Australian Preventative Health Taskforce.

Gregg, E. W., Cheng, Y. J., Cadwell, B. L., Imperatore, G., Williams, D. E., Flegal, K. M., Narayan, K. M. V. and Williamson, D. F. (2005) 'Secular trends in cardiovascular disease risk factors according to body mass index in US adults', *Journal of the American Medical Association*, 293, 15: 1868–1874.

Gregg, E. W. and Guralnik, J. M. (2007) 'Is disability obesity's price of longevity?', *Journal of The American Medical Association*, 298, 17: 2066–2067.

Gutiérrez-Fisac, J. L., Guallar-Castillón, P., Díez-Gañán, L., García, E. L., Banegas, J. R. B. and Artalejo, F. R. (2002) 'Work-related physical activity is not associated with body mass index and obesity', *Obesity Research* 10, 4: 270–276.

Halpern, S. A. (2004) 'Medical authority and the culture of rights', *Journal of Health Politics, Policy and Law* 29, 4–5: 835–852.

Halse, C. (2009) 'Bio-citizenship: virtue discourses and the birth of the bio-citizen', in J. Wright and V. Harwood (eds) *Biopolitics and the 'Obesity Epidemic': Governing Bodies*, New York: Routledge: 45–59.

Halse, C., Honey, A. and Boughtwood, D. (2007) 'The paradox of virtue: (re)thinking deviance, anorexia and schooling', *Gender and Education* 19, 2: 219–235.

Harac, L. (2008) 'School snacks under attack', *PTO Today: Helping Parent Leaders Make Great Schools*. Online. Available at: http://www.ptotoday.com/pto-today-articles/article/311-school-snacks-under-attack (accessed 18 March 2010).

Harris, K. C., Kuramoto, L. K., Schulzer, M. and Retallack, J. E. (2009) 'Effect of school-based physical activity interventions on body mass index in children: a meta-analysis', *Canadian Medical Association Journal* 180, 7: 719–726.

Harwood, V. (2009) 'Theorizing biopedagogies', in J. Wright and V. Harwood (eds) *Biopolitics and the 'Obesity Epidemic': Governing Bodies*, New York: Routledge.

Haskins, R. (2005) 'The school lunch lobby', *Education Next* 5, 3: Online. Available at: http://educationnext.org/the-school-lunch-lobby/ (accessed 18 March 2010).

Health Survey for England. (2008a) *Volume1: Physical activity and fitness*. NHS Information Centre.

Health Survey for England. (2008b) *Physical activity and fitness: Summary of key findings*. NHS Information Centre.

Heitmann, B. L., Strøger, U., Mikkelsen, K. L., Holst, C. and Sørensen, T. I. A. (2004)

'Large heterogeneity of the obesity epidemic in Danish adults', *Public Health Nutrition* 7, 3: 453–460.

Hellmich, N. (2010) 'Michelle Obama to launch initiative to fight child obesity', *USA Today*. Online. Available at: http://www.usatoday.com/news/health/weightloss/2010-01-20-michelle-obama-obesity_N.htm (accessed 18 March 2010).

Hendry, J. (2010) 'Physically fit students do better academically too: Study', *Reuters Health*. Online. Available at: http://www.reuters.com/article/idUSTRE61P08T20100226 (accessed 18 March 2010).

Hill, J. O. and Peters, J. C. (1998) 'Environmental contributions to the obesity epidemic', *Science* 280, 5368: 1371–1374.

Howell, J. and Ingham, A. (2001) 'From social problem to personal issue: the language of lifestyle', *Cultural Studies* 15, 2: 326–351.

Jackson-Leach R. and Lobstein T. (2006) 'Estimated burden of paediatric obesity and co-morbidities in Europe. Part 1. The increase in the prevalence of child obesity in Europe is itself increasing', *International Journal of Pediatric Obesity* 1, 1: 26–32.

James, W. P. (2008) 'The epidemiology of obesity: the size of the problem', *Journal of Internal Medicine* 263, 4: 336–352.

Jebb, S. (2009) 'Piling on the pounds', *Business Voice*, October: 50.

Johns Hopkins School of Public Health. (2006) 'Childhood obesity projected to increase dramatically by 2010'. Online. Available at: http://www.jhsph.edu/publichealthnews/articles/2006/wang_obesity.html (accessed 17 March 2010).

Johns, G. (2010) 'Too fat?', *New Zealand Listener*, 23–29 January: 21–23.

Johnson, A. (2001) 'Weight of a nation', *Marie Claire*, March: 233–236.

Jutel, A. (2001) 'Does size really matter? Weight and values in public health', *Perspectives in Biology and Medicine* 44, 2: 283–296.

Jutel, A. (2005) 'Weighing health: the moral burden of obesity', *Social Semiotics* 15, 2: 113–125.

Jutel, A. (2006) 'The emergence of overweight as a disease entity: measuring up normality', *Social Science and Medicine* 63, 9: 2268–2276.

Jutel, A. (2009) 'Doctor's orders: diagnosis, medical authority and the exploitation of the fat body', in J. Wright and V. Harwood (eds) Biopolitics and the 'Obesity Epidemic': Governing Bodies, New York: Routledge: 60–77.

Kassirer, J. P. and Angell, M. (1998) 'Lose weight – an ill fated new-year's resolution', *The New England Journal of Medicine* 338, 1: 52–54.

Katzmarzyk, P. T. and Ardern, C. I. (2004) 'Overweight and obesity mortality trends in Canada, 1985–2000', *Canadian Journal of Public Health* 95, 1: 16–20.

Katzmarzyk, P. T. and Mason, C. (2006) 'Prevalence of class I, II and III obesity in Canada', *Canadian Medical Association Journal* 174, 2: 156–157.

Katzmarzyk, P. T, Janssen, I. and Ardern, C. I. (2003) 'Physical inactivity, excess adiposity and premature mortality', *Obesity Reviews* 4, 4: 257–290.

Kelly, T., Yang, W., Chen, C. S., Reynolds, K. and He, J. (2008) 'Global burden of obesity in 2005 and projections to 2030', *International Journal of Obesity* 32, 9: 1431–1437.

Kennedy, E. T., Bowman, S. A. and Powell, R. (1999) 'Dietary-fat intake in the US population', *Journal of the American College of Nutrition* 18, 3: 207–212.

Knoll, C. (2008) 'State fitness scores edge up: Still, only one third of the state's students are in the healthy zone', *Los Angeles Times*. Online. Available at: http://articles.latimes.com/2008/nov/26/local/me-fitness26 (accessed 14 July 2009).

Kolata, G. (2007) *Rethinking Thin: The New Science of Weight Loss and the Myths and Realities of Dieting*, New York: Farrar, Straus, and Giroux.

Kvicala, J. (2003) 'Americans experiencing "pandemic of obesity," says Director of Centers For Disease Control And Prevention In Atlanta', *Terry College of Business*. Online. Available at: http://www.terry.uga.edu/news/releases/2003/gerberding.html (accessed 25 November 2009).

Lang, T. and Rayner, G. (2007) 'Overcoming policy cacophony on obesity: an ecological public health framework for policymakers', *Obesity Reviews* 8, 1(suppl): 165–181.

Le Fanu, J. (2000). *The Rise and Fall of Modern Medicine*, New York: Carroll and Graf.

Leichter, H. M. (2003) "Evil habits" and "personal choices": assigning responsibility for health in the 20th century', *The Milbank Quarterly* 81, 4: 603–626.

Levitt, S. D. and Dubner, S. J. (2005) *Freakonomics: A Rogue Economist Explores the Hidden Side of Everything*, New York: Harper Collins

Lioret, S., Touvier, M., Dubuisson, C., Dufour, A., Calamassi-Tran, G., Lafay, L., Volatier, J. L. and Maire, B. (2009) 'Trends in child overweight rates and energy intake in France from 1999 to 2007: relationships with socioeconomic status', *Obesity* 17, 5: 1092–1100.

Lissner, L., Björkelund, C., Heitmann, B. L., Lapidus, L., Bjorntorp, P. and Bengtsson, C. (1998) 'Secular increases in waist–hip ratio among Swedish women', *International Journal of Obesity and Related Metabolic Disorders* 22, 11: 1116–1120.

Lloyd, G. (1984) *The Man of Reason: 'Male' and 'Female' in Western Philosophy*, London: Metheun and Co.

Lobstein, T., Baur, L. and Uauy, R. (2004) 'Obesity in children and young people: a crisis in public health', *Obesity Reviews* 5 (suppl. 1): 4–85.

Lobstein, T. J., James, W. P. T. and Cole, T. J. (2003) 'Increasing levels of excess weight among children in England', *International Journal of Obesity* 27, 9: 1136–1138.

Loeb, L. (2009) 'Comment: Childhood obesity: the law's response to the surgeon general's call to action to prevent and decrease overweight and obesity', *Journal of Health Care Law and Policy* 12, 2: 295.

Louderback, L. (1970) *Fat Power*, New York: Hawthorn Books.

Ludwig, D. S. (2007) 'Childhood obesity – the shape of things to come', *New England Journal of Medicine*, 357, 23: 2325–2327.

Ludwig, D. S. and Brownell, K. D. (2003) 'Severe acute apathy syndrome', *The Boston Globe*, 29 May: A13.

Lupton, D. (1995) *The Imperative of Health: Public Health and the Regulated Body*, London: Sage.

Maine, M. (2000) *Body Wars: Making Peace With Women's Bodies*, Carlsbad: Gürze Books.

Marini, R. (2004) '"Super-sized solutions": These strategies fit outside the obesity box', *San Antonio Express-News*, 26 April: 1C.

Marks, V. (2005a) 'Healthy eating', in S. Feldman and V. Marks (eds) *Panic Nation: Unpicking The Myths We're Told About Food And Health*, London: John Blake: 43–51.

Marks, V. (2005b) 'Obesity', in S. Feldman and V. Marks (eds) *Panic Nation: Unpicking The Myths We're Told About Food And Health*, London: John Blake: 53–60.

Mason, G. (2005) 'Obesity bursting boomers' expectation of having a healthy lifestyle, expert warns', *The Globe and Mail*, 29 September: A13.

Masters, C. (2007) 'Working mums have fat kids', *News.com.au*. Online. Available at: http://www.news.com.au/features/working-mums-have-fat-kids/story-e6frfl49-1111112814233 (accessed 11 October 2009).

Mayer, V. F. (1983) 'The fat illusion', in L. Schoenfielder and B. Wieser (eds) *Shadow on a Tightrope: Writings by Women on Fat Oppression*, San Francisco: Spinsters/Aunt Lute: 3–14.

McCarron, P., Davey Smith, G. and Okasha, M. (2002) 'Secular changes in blood pressure in childhood, adolescence and young adulthood: systematic review of trends from 1948 to 1998', *Journal Of Human Hypertension* 16, 10: 677–689.

McGinnis, J. M. and Foege, W. H. (1993) 'Actual causes of death in the United States', *Journal of the American Medical Association* 270, 18: 2207–2212.

McPherson, K., Brown, M., Marsh, T. and Byatt, T. (2009) *Obesity: Recent trends in children aged 2–11y and 12–19y: Analysis from the Health Survey for England 1993–2007*, National Heart Forum.

McPherson, K., Marsh, T. and Brown M. (2007) *Foresight Tackling Obesity: Future Choices - Modelling Future Trends in Obesity and their impact on Health*: Government Office for Science.

McQueen, H. (2001) *The Essence of Capitalism: The Origins of Our Future*, Sydney: Sceptre.

Ministry of Health. (2008) *A Portrait of Health: Key Results of the 2006/07 New Zealand Health Survey*, Wellington: Ministry of Health.

Minnesota Department of Education. (2008) *Parents Are You a Fitkid Role Model? Teachers Are You a Fitkid Role Model?*. Online. Available at: https://fns.state.mn.us/StrategicPlan/PDF/ToolKit/AdutlsNutriRoleModel.pdf (accessed 25 November 2009).

Mississippi Legislature. (2007) *Senate Bill 2369: As Sent to Governor*. Online. Available at: http://www.healthyschoolsms.org/ohs_main/documents/senatebill2369.pdf (accessed 18 March 2010).

Mitchell, R. T., McDougall, C. M. and Crum, J. E. (2007) 'Decreasing prevalence of obesity in primary schoolchildren', *Archives of Disease in Childhood* 92, 2: 153–154.

Mokdad, A. H., Marks, J. S., Stroup, D. F. and Gerberding, J. L. (2004) 'Actual causes of death in the United States, 2000', *Journal of the American Medical Association* 291, 10: 1238–1245.

Monaghan, L. F. (2007) 'McDonaldizing men's bodies? Slimming, associated (ir)rationalities and resistances', *Body and Society* 13, 2: 67–93.

Monoghan, L. F. (2008) *Men and the War on Obesity: A Sociological Study*, London: Routledge.

Morris, D. (1967) *The Naked Ape*, London: Jonathan Cape.

Murphy, C. (2007) 'A bad year to be fat', *BBC Online*. Online. Available at: http://news.bbc.co.uk/1/hi/health/7140844.stm (accessed 25 December 2007).

Murray, S. (2008) *The 'Fat' Female Body*, Basingstoke: Palgrave Macmillan.

Murray, S. (2009) Marked as 'pathological': 'fat' bodies as virtual confessors. Biopolitics and the obesity epidemic: Governing Bodies. J. Wright and V. Harwood. New York, Routledge: 78–90.

Nader, P. R., Stone, E. J., Lytle, L. A., Perry, C. L., Osganian, S. K., Kelder, S., Webber, L. S., Elder, J. P., Montgomery, D., Feldman, H. A., Wu, M., Johnson, C., Parcel, G. S. and Luepker, R. V. (1999) 'Three-year maintenance of improved diet and physical activity: the CATCH cohort', *Archives of Pediatrics and Adolescent Medicine* 153, 7: 695–704.

National Alliance for Nutrition and Activity. (2005) *Model Local Wellness Policies on Physical Activity and Nutrition*. Online. Available at: http://www.schoolwellnesspolicies.org/resources/NANAWellnessPolicies.pdf accessed 30 March 2010).

National Association for Sport and Physical Education. (2010) 'Is it physical education or physical activity?'. Online. Available at: http://www.aahperd.org/naspe/publications/teachingTools/PAvsPE.cfm (accessed 30 March 2010).

National Center for Health Statistics. (2009) *Health, United States, 2008*, Hyattsville, MD: National Center for Health Statistics.

National Conference of State Legislators. (2010) *Child Obesity: 2009 Update of Legislative Policy Options*. Online. Available at: http://www.ncsl.org/?tabid=19776#Physical_ Activity (accessed 30 March 2010.)

National School Boards Association. (2000) *Fit, Healthy and Ready to Learn: A School Health Policy Guide*. Online. Available at: http://www.nsba.org/MainMenu/ SchoolHealth/SearchSchoolHealth/FitHealthyandReadytoLearnPartIASchoolHealthPol icyGuide.aspx (accessed 18 March 2010).

Nestle, M. (2000) 'Obese? Food firms say "eat more"', *Deseret News*, 29 June: A19.

Nestle, M. (2002a) *Food Politics: How the Food Industry Influences Nutrition and Health*, Berkeley, California: University of California Press.

Nestle, M. (2002b) Profit drive requires force-feeding the fat, *The Times Higher*, 15 March: 16–17.

Newman, M. (2006) 'Soda distributors to end most school sales,' *The New York Times*. Online. Available at: http://www.nytimes.com/2006/05/03/health/03cnd-soda.html?_ r=2&hp&ex=1146715200&en=88adf9b55e9c8710&ei=5094&partner=homepage (accessed 18 March 2010).

New York State Department of Education. (2010) *New York Certification Requirements*. Online. Available at: http://www.emsc.nysed.gov/ciai/pe/peqa.html (accessed 18 March 2010).

Nordqvist, C. (2006) 'Obesity rates among American women falling', *Medical News Today*. Online. Available at: http://www.medicalnewstoday.com/articles/41048.php (accessed 3 February 2009).

Norton, K., Dollman, J., Martin, M. and Harten, N. (2006) 'Descriptive epidemiology of childhood overweight and obesity in Australia: 1901–2003', *International Journal of Pediatric Obesity* 1, 4: 232–238.

O'Connor-Fleming, M. L. and Parker, E. (2001). *Health Promotion: Principles and Practice in the Australian Context*, Crows Nest, NSW: Allen and Unwin.

Office of Healthy Schools. (2008) *Frequently Asked Questions*. Online. Available at: http:// www.healthyschoolsms.org/nutrition_services/faqvend.htm#vend4 (accessed 18 March 2010).

Ogden, C. L., Carroll, M. D., Curtin, L. R., Lamb, M. M. and Flegal, K. M. (2010) 'Prevalence of high body mass index in US children and adolescents, 2007–2008', *Journal of the American Medical Association* 303, 3: 242–249.

Ogden, C. L., Carroll, M. D., Curtin, L. R., McDowell, M. A., Tabak, C. J. and Flegal, K. M. (2006) 'Prevalence of overweight and obesity in the United States, 1999–2004', *Journal of the American Medical Association* 295, 13: 1549–1555.

Ogden, C. L., Carroll, M. D. and Flegal, K. M. (2008) 'High Body Mass Index for age among US children and adolescents, 2003–2006', *Journal of the American Medical Association* 299, 20: 2401–2405.

Ogden, C. L., Carroll, M. D., McDowell, M. A. and Flegal, K. M. (2007) 'Obesity among adults in the United States—no change since 2003–2004', *NCHS data brief no 1*, Hyattsville, MD: National Center for Health Statistics.

Ohio Department of Education. (2010) 'Frequently asked questions about the physical education graduation requirements'. Online. Available at: http://www.ode.state.oh.us/ GD/Templates/Pages/ODE/ODEDetail.aspx?page=3&TopicRelationID=1690&Conten tID=45762&Content=79827 (accessed 30 March 2010).

Olds, T. S., Tomkinson, G. R., Ferrar, K. E. and Maher, C. A. (2010) 'Trends in the prevalence of childhood overweight and obesity in Australia between 1985 and 2008', *International Journal of Obesity* 34, 1: 57–66.

Oliver, J. E. (2006) *Fat Politics: The Real Story Behind America's Obesity Epidemic*, Oxford: Oxford University Press.

Olshansky, S. J., Passaro, D. J., Hershow, R. C., Layden, J., Carnes, B. A., Brody, J., Hayflick, L., Butler, R. N., Allison, D. B. and Ludwig, D. S. (2005) 'A potential decline in life expectancy in the United States in the 21st century', *New England Journal of Medicine* 352, 11: 1138–1145.

Orpana, H. M., Berthelot, J. M., Kaplan, M. S., Feeny, D. H., McFarland, B. and Ross, N. A. (2010) BMI and mortality: results from a national longitudinal study of Canadian adults, *Obesity* 18, 1: 214–218.

Péneau, S., Salanave, B., Maillard-Teyssier, L., Rolland-Cachera, M. F., Vergnaud, A. C., Méjean, C., Czernichow, S., Vol, S., Tichet, J., Castetbon, K. and Hercberg, S. (2009) 'Prevalence of overweight in 6- to 15-year-old children in central/western France from 1996 to 2006: trends toward stabilization', *International Journal of Obesity* 33, 4: 401–407.

Perkins, B. K. and Piñeyro, C. J. (2009) 'From the National School Boards Association', *American School Board Journal*, February: 32.

Peterbaugh, J. S. (2009) 'The emperor's tailors: the failure of the medical weight loss paradigm and its causal role in the obesity of America', *Diabetes, Obesity and Metabolism* 11, 6: 557–570.

Phillips, A. (2009) 'Let there be baked goods: Students begin to fight back against new bake sale rules,' *Gotham Schools*. Online. Available at: http://gothamschools.org/2009/10/12/students-begin-to-fight-back-against-new-bake-sale-rules/ (accessed 18 March 2010).

Pietinen, P., Vartiainen, E. and Männistö, S. (1996) 'Trends in body mass index and obesity among adults in Finland from 1972 to 1992', *International Journal of Obesity and Related Metabolic Disorders* 20, 2: 114–120.

Porter, R. (2002) *Blood and Guts: A Short History of Medicine*, New York: W. W. Norton & Company.

Prime Minister of Australia. (2009) Transcript of interview with Kevin Rudd on radio station 3AW's Neil Mitchell program. Online. Available at: http://www.pm.gov.au/node/6175 (accessed 11 December 2009).

Raghuwanshi, M., Kirschner, M., Xenachis, C., Ediale, K. and Amir, J. (2001) 'Treatment of morbid obesity in inner-city women', *Obesity Research* 9, 6: 342–347.

Ralston, K., Newman, C., Clauson, A., Guthrie, J., and Buzby, J. (2008) 'The National School Lunch Program: Background, trends and issues', *Economic Research Report*, 61: i–48. Online. Available at: http://www.ers.usda.gov/Publications/ERR61/ERR61.pdf (accessed 18 March 2010).

Rana, C., Herman, V. O. and Stefaan, D. (2009) 'Trends in social inequalities in obesity: Belgium, 1997 to 2004', *Preventive Medicine* 48, 1: 54–58.

Reed, E. (1976) *Sexism and Science*, New York: Pathfinder Press.

Reich, C. A. (1970) *The Greening of America*, New York: Random House.

Research Update. (2009) 'New direction needed for obesity research, Deakin health expert claims', *Deakin University*. Online. Available at: http://www.gsdm.com.au/newsletters/deakin/june09/16.html (accessed 12 June 2009).

Rice, C. (2007) 'Becoming "the fat girl": acquisition of an unfit identity', *Women's Studies International Forum*, 30, 2: 158–174.

Rich, E. and Evans, J. (2009) 'Performative health in schools: welfare policy, neoliberalism and social regulation?', in J. Wright and V. Harwood (eds) *Biopolitics and the 'Obesity Epidemic': Governing Bodies*, New York: Routledge.

Rich, E., Holroyd, R. and Evans, J. (2004) 'Hungry to be noticed': young women, anorexia and schooling. *Body Knowledge and Control: Studies in the Sociology of Physical Education and Health*. J. Evans, B. Davies and J. Wright. London, Routledge: 173–190.

Riskworld.com. (1999) 'New study finds obesity costs over $200 Billion; obesity tied to costly chronic illnesses that make medical bills skyrocket'. Online. Available at: http://www.riskworld.com/PressRel/1999/PR99aa85.htm (accessed 10 April 2008).

Robert Wood Johnson Foundation. (2009) *Mediocre Grades for School Wellness Policies: Landmark Study Pinpoints the Shortcomings, Poor Enforcement of Nutrition and Activity Guidelines*. Online. Available at: http://www.rwjf.org/childhoodobesity/product.jsp?id=46308 (accessed 7 April 2010).

Robison, J. and Carrier, K. (2004) *The Spirit and Science of Holistic Health*, Bloomington: AuthorHouse.

Rodgers, E. (2008) 'Obesity figures staggering: Roxon', *ABC*. Online. Available at: http://www.abc.net.au/news/stories/2008/06/20/2280723.htm (accessed 20 June 2008).

Romero-Corral, A., Montori, V. M., Somers, V. K., Korinek, J., Thomas, R. J., Allison, T. G., Mookadam, F. and Lopez-Jimenez, F. (2006) 'Association of bodyweight with total mortality and with cardiovascular events in coronary artery disease: a systematic review of cohort studies', *The Lancet*, 368, 9536: 666–678.

Romon, M., Lommez, A., Tafflet, M., Basdevant, A., Oppert, J. M., Bresson, J. L., Ducimetière, P., Charles, M. A. and Borys, J. M. (2008) 'Downward trends in the prevalence of childhood overweight in the setting of 12-year school- and community-based programmes', *Public Health Nutrition* 12, 10: 1735–1742.

Rumbach, D. (2006) 'Aerobics little help for weight: America's fitness era hasn't stemmed obesity explosion', *South Bend Tribune*, 18 October.

Rumbelow, H. (2009) 'Exercise? A fat lot of good that is for weight loss', *Times Online*. Online. Available at: http://women.timesonline.co.uk/tol/life_and_style/women/diet_and_fitness/article6878496.ece (accessed 20 October 2009).

Salanave, B., Peneau, S., Rolland-Cachera, M. F., Hercberg, S. and Castetbon, K. (2009) 'Stabilization of overweight prevalence in French children between 2000 and 2007', *International Journal of Pediatric Obesity* 4, 2: 66–72.

Schulte, B. (2006) 'Once just a sweet birthday treat, the cupcake becomes a cause', *The Washington Post*. Online. Available at: http://www.washingtonpost.com/wp-dyn/content/article/2006/12/10/AR2006121001008.html (accessed 18 March 2010).

ScienceDaily. (2009) 'Sedentary lives can be deadly: physical inactivity poses greatest health risk to Americans, expert say'. Online. Available at: http://www.sciencedaily.com/releases/2009/08/090810024825.htm (accessed 10 December 2009).

Schlesinger, M. (2002) 'A loss of faith: the sources of reduced political legitimacy for the American medical profession', *The Milbank Quarterly* 80, 2: 185–235

Schlosser, E. (2001) *Fast Food Nation: What the All-American Meal is Doing to the World*, London: Allen Lane.

Scottish Government. (2005) *The Scottish Health Survey 2003: Volume 3: Children*, Edinburgh: Scottish Government.

Scottish Government. (2009) *The Scottish Health Survey: Volume 1: Main Report*, Edinburgh: Scottish Government.

Sharma, A. J., Grummer-Strawn, L. M., Dalenius, K., Galuska, D., Anandappa, M., Borland, E., Mackintosh, H. and Smith, R. (2009) 'Obesity prevalence among low-income, preschool-aged children – United States, 1998–2008', *Mortality and Morbidity Weekly Report* 58, 28: 769–773.

Simon, M. (2006) *Appetite for Profit: How the Food Industry Undermines our Health and How to Fight Back*, New York: Nation Books.

Simpson, J. A., MacInnis, R. J., Peeters, A., Hopper, J. L., Giles, G. G. and English, D. R. (2007) 'A comparison of adiposity measures as predictors of all-cause mortality: The Melbourne Collaborative Cohort Study', *Obesity* 15, 4: 994–1003.

Sjöberg, A., Lissner, L., Albertsson-Wikland, K. and Mårild, S. (2008) 'Recent anthropometric trends among Swedish school children: evidence for decreasing prevalence of overweight in girls', *Acta Paediatrica* 97, 1: 118–123.

Sky News. (2009) 'Turn off the TV and play dodgeball instead'. Online. Available at: http://news.sky.com/skynews/Home/UK-News/Child-Obesity-British-Heart-Foundation-Launches-Dodgeball-Challenge-In-UK-Schools/Article/200909415393686?f=rss (accessed 10 January 2010).

Smith, J. (2005) 'EU food industry called to battle against obesity', *Reuters Health E-Line*, 25 January.

Social Issues Research Centre. (2005) *Obesity and the Facts: An Analysis of Data from the Health Survey for England 2003*, Oxford: Social Issues Research Centre.

Social Issues Research Centre. (2006a) *The Impact of Sport on the Workplace*, Oxford: Social Issues Research Centre.

Social Issues Research Centre. (2006b) *Fattened statistics*, Oxford: Social Issues Research Centre.

Snow, T. (2007) 'Can nurses tackle the obesity crisis', *Nursing Standard* 22, 3: 12–13.

South Carolina Band Director's Association. (n.d.) 'High school marching bands: "the sport of the arts". Online. Available at: http://www.scbda.org/PECredit/PositionsStatement-PECredit.htm (accessed 18 March 2010).

Stamatakis, E., Primatesta, P., Chinn, S., Rona, R. and Falascheti, E. (2005) 'Overweight and obesity trends from 1974 to 2003 in English children: what is the role of socioeconomic factors?', *Archives of Disease in Childhood* 90, 10: 999–1004.

Stanton, R. (2009) 'Who will take responsibility for obesity in Australia?', *Public Health* 123, 3: 280–282.

Starky, S. (2005) *The Obesity Epidemic in Canada*. Parliamentary Information and Research Service.

Stearns, P. N. (1997). *Fat History: Bodies and Beauty in the Modern West*, New York: New York University Press.

Stein, R. (2004) 'CDC study overestimated deaths from obesity', *Washington Post*, 24 November: A11.

Stewart, S. T., Cutler, D. M. and Rosen, A. B. (2009) 'Forecasting the effects of obesity and smoking on U.S. life expectancy', *New England Journal of Medicine* 361, 23: 2252–2260.

Strand, B. and Sommer, C. (2005) 'Should marching band be allowed to replace physical education credits? An analysis', *Physical Educator* 62, 3: 164–168.

Sundblom, E., Petzold, M., Rasmussen, F., Callmer, E. and Lissner, L. (2008) 'Childhood overweight and obesity prevalences levelling off in Stockholm but socioeconomic differences persist', *International Journal of Obesity* 32, 10: 1525–1530.

Swinburn, B. (2008) 'Obesity prevention: the role of policies, laws and regulations', *Australia and New Zealand Health Policy* 5:12 doi:10.1186/1743-8462-5-12.

Tenzer, S. (1989) 'Fat acceptance therapy (F. A. T.): a non-dieting group approach to physical wellness, insight and self-acceptance', in L. S. Brown and E. D. Rothblum (eds) *Fat Oppression and Psychotherapy: A Feminist Perspective*, New York: The Haworth Press: 39–47.

Teutsch, D. (2003) 'Kids pay a heavy price for lifestyle', *The Sun-Herald*, 5 January: 25.

Thacker, B. (2004) *The Naked Man Festival and Other Excuses to Fly Around the World*, Crows Nest, NSW: Allen and Unwin.

The Obesity Society. (2009) 'What is obesity'. Online. Available at: http://www.obesity. org/information/what_is_obesity.asp (accessed 14 December 2009).

Thompson, J. L. (2008) 'Obesity and consequent health risks: is prevention realistic and achievable?', *Archives of Disease in Childhood* 93, 9: 722–724.

Thone, R. R. (1997) *Fat – A Fate Worse Than Death? Women, Weight, and Appearance*, New York: The Harrington Park Press.

Tiger, L. (1999) *The Decline of Males: The First Look at an Unexpected New World for Men and Women*, New York: St. Martin's Press.

Trost, S. (2006) 'Public health and physical education', in D. Kirk, D. Macdonald and M. O'Sullivan (eds) *Handbook of Physical Education*, London: Sage: 163–187.

Tverdal, A. (1996) 'Høyde, vekt og kroppsmasseindeks for menn og kvinner i aldermen 40–42 år [Height, weight and body mass index of men and women aged 40–42 years]', *Tidsskrift for den Norske Lægeforening* 116: 2152–2156.

Unified School District #232. (2010) *Winning with Wellness*. Online. Available at: http:// www.usd232.org/education/dept/dept.php?sectiondetailid=14443& (accessed 18 March 2010).

United States Department of Health and Human Services. (2004) 'The growing epidemic of childhood obesity', *Testimony to the The Subcommittee on Competition, Infrastructure and Foreign Commerce, Science, and Transportation, March 2, 2004*. Online. Available at: http://www.hhs.gov/asl/testify/t040302.html (accessed 20 November 2009).

Vander Schee, C. (2004) 'The privatization of food services in schools: Undermining children's health, social equity, and democratic education', in D. Boyles (ed.) *Schools or Markets?: Commercialism, Privatization, and School-business Partnerships*, New York: Lawrence Erlbaum: 1–30.

Vander Schee, C. (2008) 'The politics of health as a school-sponsored ethic: Foucault, neoliberalism, and the unhealthy employee' *Educational Policy* 22, 6: 854–874.

Walker, A. R. P. (2003) 'The obesity pandemic. Is it beyond control?', *Journal of the Royal Society for the Promotion of Health* 123, 3: 150–151.

Wang, Y. and Beydoun, M. A. (2007) 'The obesity epidemic in the United States - gender, age, socioeconomic, racial/ethnic, and geographic characteristics: a systematic review and meta-regression analysis', *Epidemiologic Reviews* 29, 1: 6–28.

Wang, Y., Beydoun, M. A., Liang, L. Caballero, B. and Kumanyika S. K. (2008) 'Will all Americans become overweight or obese? Estimating the progression and cost of the US obesity epidemic', *Obesity* 16, 10: 2323–2330.

Wann, M. (1998) *Fat? So? Because You Don't Have to Apologize for Your Size*, Berkley, California: Ten Speed Press.

Wen, L. M., Orr, N., Millett, C. and Rissel, C. (2006) 'Driving to work and overweight and obesity: findings from the 2003 New South Wales Health Survey, Australia, *International Journal of Obesity* 30, 5: 782–786.

Wilson, R. (2009) 'College employees lose weight, and privacy in campus wellness programs', *Chronicle of Higher Education,* LVI, 16. Online. Available at: http://chronicle. texterity.com/chronicle/20091211a/?pg=1 (accessed 18 March 2010).

Wolff, H., Delhumeau, C., Beer-Borst, S., Golay, A., Costanza, M. C. and Morabia, A. (2006) 'Converging prevalences of obesity across educational groups in Switzerland', *Obesity* 14, 11: 2080–2088.

Wooley, S. C. and Garner, D. M. (1991) 'Obesity treatment: the high cost of false hope', *Journal of the American Dietetic Association* 91, 10: 1248–1251.

World Health Organization. (2008) *School Policy Framework: Implementation of the WHO Global Strategy on Diet, Physical Activity and Health.* Online. Available at: http://www. who.int/dietphysicalactivity/SPF-en-2008.pdf (accessed 18 March 2010).

YRBSS. (2009) 'Trends in the Prevalence of Obesity, Dietary Behaviors, and Weight Control Practices National YRBS: 1991–2007'. Online. Available at: http://www.cdc. gov/HealthyYouth/yrbs/trends.htm (accessed 10 December 2009).

Zaninotto, P., Wardle, H., Stamatakis, E., Mindell, J. and Head, J. (2006) *Forecasting Obesity to 2010*: National Centre for Social Research.

Zanker, C. and Gard, M. (2008) 'Fatness, fitness and the moral universe of sport and physical activity', *Sociology of Sport Journal* 25, 1: 48–65.

Zimmet, P. and Jennings, G. (2008) 'Curbing the obesity epidemic', *The Age*. Online. Available at: http://www.theage.com.au/news/opinion/curbing-the-obesity-epidemic/ 2008/02/21/1203467280758.html (accessed 7 March 2009).

Index